CW00787160

Researching Women's Health:
Methods and Process

Researching Women's Health: *Methods and Process*

Edited by
L McKie

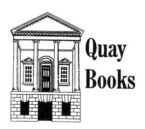

Quay
Books

Quay Books, Division of Mark Allen Publishing Limited
Jesses Farm, Snow Hill, Dinton, Nr Salisbury, Wilts, SP3 5HN

© Mark Allen Publishing Ltd, 1996

British Library Cataloguing-in-Publication Data
A catalogue record for this book is available from the British
Library

ISBN 1-85642-089 2

All rights reserved. No part of this material may be reproduced,
stored in a retrieval system, or transmitted in any form, or by any
means, electrical, mechanical, photographic, recording, or
otherwise, without the prior permission of the publishers.

Printed and bound in Great Britain by
Biddles Ltd, Guildford and King's Lynn

CONTENTS

Acknowledgements

Many people have assisted in the composition of this text. We cannot name everyone individually but would like to extend particular thanks to:

- the participants in the research projects presented in Part Two

- Natalie Aird who assisted with the early stages of editing

- Valery Moran of Quay Publishing for her ongoing support and editorial advice

As with any creative project the process took time and made demands upon our friends and families. Thanks to all those who took on additional domestic work and those who listened as we mused on the ideas included in the text.

Any errors or omissions are those of the respective authors and the views expressed by authors are not necessarily those of their employing organisations.

Linda McKie
Department of General Practice
University Of Aberdeen
July 1995

LIST OF CONTRIBUTORS

Alison Bowes is Senior Lecturer in Sociology at the University of Stirling, Department of Applied Social Science, Stirling, FK9 4LA

Ruth Cochrane is Senior Registrar in Obstetrics and Gynaecology at St Mary's Hospital, Praed Street, London W2. She previously worked as a research fellow to Wendy Savage in East London where the work for this study was carried out.

Teresa Domokos is Research Fellow at the University of Stirling, Department of Applied Social Science, Stirling, FK9 4LA

Sharon Gray is founder and ex-director of Child Abuse Listening Line (CALL). She is currently Director of the Independent Training Advocacy and Counselling Service (ITACS). She is a therapist, trainer and consultant specialising in work with adults and children who have experienced sexual abuse.

Susan Gregory is research officer in the Department of Agricultural Economics at the University Of Reading, RG6 2AA

Marietta Higgs is Consultant Paediatrician at the Queen Elizabeth Hospital, Gateshead and Chair of the North East England branch of BASPCAN.

Linda McKie is Senior Lecturer in Health Education, Department of General Practice, University of Aberdeen, Foresterhill Health Centre, Westburn Road, Aberdeen, AB9 2AY

Tina Posner is Senior Research Fellow at the Centre for Mental Health Nursing Research, School of Nursing, Queensland University of Technology, Kelvin Grove Campus, Locked Bag No 2, Red Hill, Queensland 4059, Australia

Keith Pringle is Senior Lecturer in Applied Social Studies at the University of Sunderland and formerly practised as a qualified social worker for ten years.

Vicki Taylor is Health of the Nation Manager at Camden and Islington Health, 110 Hampstead Road, London, NW1 2LJ

Jane Wills is Senior Lecturer in Health Promotion, School of Education and Health Studies, University of South Bank, London, SE1 0AA.

PREFACE

This text combines a practical consideration of research methods with a critical review, by the contributors, of the process of research. It is complied and presented as a text book for nurses and those studying courses in health care and related subjects.

There has been a substantial growth in degree courses in the area of nursing and health care. Intrinsic to these courses is the study of research methods. Not only do health care workers need to comprehend research reports and the implications of such work but increasingly they are requested to conduct research both as students and as practitioners. Added to this is the introduction of the purchaser, provider relationship in the NHS which has placed an increased emphasis upon the evaluation of policy and practice. Health workers are actively involved in many such reviews.

This text aims to:

a. define the concept of research with reference to practical examples of research from projects conducted by contributors;

b. explore the process of research through the examination of projects undertaken by active researchers, and

c. suggest practical means for determining research questions, research design, evaluating the research process, writing up and disseminating projects.

The text is composed of three parts, each considering a dimension of the research process, namely:

* Part One; An Introduction to Research

* Part Two; Researching Women's Health

- Concluding Comments: Reflection and Dissemination

In Part One, the aim is to introduce research and research methods. In Chapter One 'Getting Started' consideration is given to the design of a research project and the potential approaches to research. The principles and continuum of quantitative and qualitative approaches are presented, as are feminist approaches to research and the process of action research. In Chapter Two "A Range of Methods" a number of research methods are outlined, namely, observation, discussion groups, interviews, questionnaires and the control trial. Methods of sampling are presented and the potential for multi method projects considered.

In Part Two, contributors present 'a warts and all portrait' of the reality of conducting research on women's health issues. Semi-structured interviews were employed by Wills, Bowes and Domokos, and Taylor. Wills used the interview method to explore 'Women's Experiences of Infertility', presented in Chapter Three. In Chapter Four Bowes and Domokos used the interview method in a study of Asian women's views of their health. In their chapter, entitled 'Race, Gender and Culture in South Asian Women's Health: A Study in Glasgow' they reflect upon this research method. Taylor identifies and examines 'Men's Perceptions of Pregnancy' in Chapter Five considering the issue of a woman interviewing men and the relevance of male views in the process of pregnancy and the health of women.

Questionnaires were used by Cochrane and Gray, Higgs and Pringle. In Chapter Six 'Women's Experiences of Antenatal Care in Tower Hamlets' Cochrane employed a questionnaire as a means of collecting and comparing data on women's usage and views on different types of antenatal care. Gray, Higgs and Pringle employed the questionnaire as a means of collecting data from busy professional people. In Chapter Seven, 'Services for People who have been Sexually Abused' they reflect upon the drawbacks of the method but conclude that the disadvantages outweigh the need to gain data on highly pressurised respondents.

In Chapters Eight and Nine, Gregory and McKie, and Posner present multi-method projects. Gregory and McKie conducted discussion groups prior to writing a questionnaire on women's use and views of cervical screening services. Their experiences of developing a project with a range of professional groups are presented in Chapter Eight `Negotiation and Compromise in Researching Women's Views of the Cervical Smear Test'. In Chapter Nine `Differences of Method and Aspects of Process: Researching Cervical Screening Services' Posner reports on two projects investigating women's views of cervical screening. The first project involved large scale population surveys and the second was an in-depth study of the experiences of a series of women going through medical procedures. She contrasts the methods employed.

The concluding chapter considers the process of writing up and disseminating results to a range of groups, not least the respondents. The continued importance and relevance of research in health and social services is noted. As health workers and students continue to examine health care services and health issues, the study of approaches to research and research methods is crucial to personal and career development. In addition the voices of the women and men who contributed to the studies presented in this text illuminate the experiences of those using and organising services, and in particular, illuminate the experiences of the less powerful.

Researching Women's Health: Methods and Process

Part One

An Introduction to Research

CHAPTER ONE
GETTING STARTED

Linda McKie

Introduction

Perhaps the most difficult, and certainly the most thought provoking stage of the research process, is the initial one of formulating the research question. Sometimes it is difficult to consider just one question; your interests may lie in exploring a vast topic such as palliative care. If this is the case your "research" is best considered in terms of commencing with a review of literature and available information on completed and on going research in the area. The enthusiasm of a prospective researcher can lack direction; can lack a focus that is necessary for the effective design of projects and, as a consequence, the efficient and effective conduct of research. By reflecting on the origins of a research project it is the aim of this chapter to explore:

1. the question what is research?;

2. the process of formulating a specific research question, and

3. the alternative methodologies of social and health care research.

Asking questions

As Sapsford and Abbott (1992, p3) note research can be `presented as something mysterious and technical'. In fact it is an activity central to many areas of employment and further training and education. Research is not only evident in the somewhat rarefied process of studying for further qualifications but can be an

1

extension of everyday enquiries. Why do some women choose not to participate in cervical screening services? What are the views of men on pregnancy? Should their views be considered when designing antenatal services? What do women, in inner city London, think of their local antenatal services? These are questions that any one of us, regardless of our involvement in health services, might wish to consider further. But without conducting research our answers to these questions are, invariably, based upon the anecdotal, individual experience or the outcomes of debate with others. Such information must be placed within the context of a systematic examination of the research question. For example, the practice nurse may have her own ideas why some women do not attend the health centre for a cervical smear test. But as she is unlikely to meet these women how realistic will the nurses' responses be? What is required to answer such a question is for someone to actually meet and speak with the women who do not go to the health centre for a cervical smear test.

These and many other questions concerning women's health are posed in this text. The research that seeks to answer such questions reflects a variety of approaches and research methods (for a review of research methods see Chapter Two). Research methods provide what Jones (1993, p112) terms a 'tool shed' for data collection and in Part Two of the text contributors outline the practicalities of research. But for the moment it is important to consider the initial starting point — how the research question and thus the research process — is actually framed.

What is research?

Sapsford and Abbott (1992, p4) contend that:

> *"...research tries not to take for granted what is taken for granted by common sense."*

Research attempts to apply certain rules to the exploration of questions within the reality of the everyday context. It is often conducted for an audience and not just as a component of personal research. Sapsford and Abbott (*ibid*) propose that in addition to personal research there are audiences for three types of research, namely:

a.   the evaluation of new or existing practices;

b.   the academic research, and

c.   the evaluation of professional practice.

For those working and studying in health care the evaluation of new or existing practices have become a major area of work and a main source of financial support for research. Evaluation studies are not solely concerned with outcome measures, such as how many patients used a service, what was the cost per user, how did patients assess the service, but also the process of a service or clinical intervention. The process element is concerned with the identification of all those involved and an exploration of the organisation and relationships involved in a project. Research concerned with the introduction of a new project are often termed "before and after" the project and this form of research also documents what existed prior to the introduction of a new service.

Academic research seeks to build an understanding of a service area or clinical treatment. It also examines social and economic factors which impact upon health and health care services, e.g., inequalities in health, social and psychological status. Academic research can inform policy and practice, although this is not a central focus of the research. However the general aim of building a body of knowledge in an area can usefully inform policy and practice and the researcher working in a health care setting may find a welcome audience for research conducted as part of personal study.

Evaluating professional practice can involve the assessment of your own practice or that of others and the evaluation of the impact of altering any aspect of professional practice. This type of research can be especially controversial as it can appear to be judgmental. The concept of objectivity can be an especially difficult one to ensure as any researcher, will have preconceived ideas. In this type of research it is important for the researcher to be honest and recount their conception of a particular aspect of professional research before commencing their research.

It is important to consider how the reality of research differs from the text book renditions. Research should not be perceived of as a 'scientific' process which works with research methods to a set of pre-determined rules to obtain answers (Stanley and Wise, 1993). The notion of a linear process — of moving from the question, to the choice of methods, to the collection of data, analysis and thus to an answer— is far from the reality of everyday research. The reality is as Stanley and Wise (Stanley and Wise *ibid*, p.150) suggest that what happens is "idiosyncratic and redolent with 'mistakes' and 'confusion's' ". This they contend is at the heart of research but it is a heart which is often denied by researchers keen to adhere to the supposed rules of a scientifically based research process. The reality of what is produced in many text books or journal articles is that:

"research as it is described is not research as it is experienced"
(Stanley and Wise, 1993, p.153)

The mystification of research and the research process has resulted in many feeling that research should only be carried out by the academic researcher with years of training in scientific work or research methods. Yet as noted earlier research is an extension of what happens in everyday life; an extension based upon the premise of the questions which interest the individual or group. What causes great anxiety is that the actual experience of research appears to differ from the classic text book expositions of the research process that are in themselves over simplistic and invariably misleading renditions of that very process.

It is a key component of this text that contributors have presented "a warts and all portrait" of their experience of research in the area of women's health. In discussing and writing the text the contributors all expressed the experience of personal involvement and personal investment on the part of those who responded to and those who conducted the research. Rather than hide these realities and write up their research in a manner which reproduces the sanitised versions of many reports, contributors hope that their honest portraits of research in action will encourage you to ask your question or questions and seek answers from your own or collaborative research.

The changing status of health care research

Today every Regional Health Authority, Health Board and most major care organisations have a research strategy. It appears an accepted maxim that quality research must underlie policy and service provisions. As a result of this change in attitude to research it is now an expectation that most health care practitioners and policy makers should be able to comprehend research results, assess the quality of research and potentially commission or conduct research. The driving force behind this change in status for research is both economic and politically led. Budgets are limited while patients are encouraged to express their views of care by documents such as the Patients' Charter. The service manager is left with the thorny question "what will satisfy the patient, the practitioner and auditor?" Current debates in political circles avidly reported in the media argue over the relative merits of the views of these groups and the evident power imbalance between the auditor, the practitioner and the patient. Research into both clinical and social aspects of care is perceived by many as a reasoned response to these debates.

As noted earlier, the actual conduct of research, no matter which method you consider, is likely to be flawed by, for example, problems of access to data or patients, or the introduction of additional clinical practices. So the debate can become one about "what kinds of evidence researchers and health care workers find convincing" (Daly, McDonald and Willis, 1992, p1). This debate focuses upon the rigour and appropriateness (or otherwise) of the methods employed.

Principles and approaches

Health care research is increasingly characterised by an acceptance of a range of methods, for example interviews, discussion groups and questionnaires. There has been a shift from the dominance of the experimental method and the controlled trial to methods that consider the social aspects of practice. Indeed as Newell (1992) notes the control trial can incorporate and draw upon a range of methods that can consider both clinical and social research questions.

The classic distinction drawn to define the principles of a method are whether the method is inductive or deductive. **Inductive** approaches generate analyses based upon the on-going review of data. **Qualitative** methods proceed from inductive principles by exploring issues and questions in a search for patterns. Qualitative methods can generate hypotheses. By contrast **deductive** approaches accept or reject hypotheses and methods based upon this approach are known as **quantitative** methods. A hypothesis is a provisional assumption made to investigate the logic of that very assumption, e.g., that a particular drug or surgical intervention improves a known medical condition.

Table 1: A Continuum of approaches to research and research methods

qualitative (*hypothesis-generating*)	*observation, case studies, autobiography
	*discussion groups, *interviews
	*questionnairs
	analysis of documentary sources
	analysis of official sources
	*patient-centred randomised control trials
	*randomised control trials
(*hypothesis-testing*) quantitative	longitudinal studies

Source: adopted from Najman *et al* (1992)
*denotes that the method is considered in Chapter 2

The randomised control trial is the method most closely associated with the quantitative end of the continuum. At the far end of the quantitative scale the randomised control trial is often restricted to small sample sizes and takes place in a contrived context, e.g. patients are allocated to intervention and control groups with the intervention group receiving a drug and the control group receiving a placebo. It is proposed that this method has a high validity as the hypothesis can be rejected or accepted. But this testing must be repeated as this repeated failure enhances confidence in the probable validity.

Moving back along the continuum, the questionnaire seeks to quantify information. However in composition, questionnaires may combine questions that seek to collect information (e.g., age, gender, clinic attendance) and those which aim to elicit views from which we may generate (induce) assumptions on a topic or issue.

Qualitative methods are characterised by their basis upon:

a. exploratory potential of research; assumptions are not made with regards to what is relevant to the respondents. Methods like observation and the discussion group encourage a topic or research question to be explored by the respondents;

b. explanatory means of the process; explanations arise from the respondents and the research situation with the potential for researcher bias in explanations limited by the analysis of social situations and respondents' words, and

c. descriptions of social and clinical situations and the people who work or are treated in such settings.

Qualitative methods have their origins in a range of disciplines including sociology, psychology, philosophy and social anthropology and as Jones (1993, p119) argues qualitative approaches both drew upon and challenged scientific (or positivist) research.

Much debate has been conducted as to the relative merits of quantitative or qualitative methods. The qualitative, quantitative divide is proposed here as a continuum over which research methods range. Multi-method projects draw upon two or more methods and may well combine qualitative and quantitative approaches.

Feminist perspectives on researching women's health

Feminism has as its purpose to understand the oppression women experience so this might be challenged. Feminists are both a part of the process of discovery and feminist researchers are responsible for attempting to illuminate oppression and create change.

At the heart of this approach to research is the concept of illumination; of illuminating the lives of the oppressed and those involved in and maintaining the mechanisms of discrimination

(Stanley and Wise, 1993). Given the high proportion of women working in health care professions (Witz, 1992), experiencing health care (Roberts, 1990; Roberts, 1992) and the evident inequality in women's lives (Oakley, 1993) it is not surprising that a feminist approach to research receives growing interest and support. Increasingly researchers are also beginning to illuminate the lives of men and the relationship between male experiences of working in health care and being in receipt of health services, as patients or relatives of patients. This work adds a further dimension to the study of oppression.

A distinct range of feminist methods does not exist. Rather a feminist approach can be identified. Feminists may adopt any one of the methods cited earlier in table one. But it is in the principles which infuse the design of projects and the application of the methods that a feminist approach can be identified. These principles can be cited as:

a.   a recognition of the impact of any research upon respondents and the researcher;

b.   recognising the responsibility of this impact and the potential parallels in experience between women as the researcher and researched. This necessitates an empathy and emotion in both the conduct and dissemination of the research. As a consequence emotion, expressed and experienced acquires a status in research often denied in so-called "scientific" approaches and methods;

c.   the concepts of objectivity and subjectivity are not strictly set in contrast to each other but are defined in terms of the contradictions, contrasts and parallels evident as the researcher and researched work through the research process;

d.   also evident is the method of autobiography, of both the researcher and researched writing about their experiences of the research and feeding those into the process of research and research results, and

e. issues concerning power and authority surrounding the research, both evident in practice and documentation are considered.

A feminist approach to research is characterised by its incorporation of the totality of human experience, emotion and values in the data collection. Also it is an approach characterised by a concern for ethics; for the "moral choices between things and actions seen as good or bad" (Stanley and Wise, 1993, p200). A feminist ethic brings together the basic concern for oppression and the practical conduct of human relationships within the research process, together with a consideration of the relationship between all involved in the research process and research context.

Action research

Action research is an approach to research in which the researcher feeds on giving results back to service providers or organisers. Action research often combines a range of methods and is a process of working which does not wait until the end of a project to feed back results but documents ongoing activities and changes, feeding this information into service working and research. In this process, it is important to identify anything that might cause change or impact upon service delivery. Participation of the researcher is central and that participation can act as a model for patient involvement in a service.

It can be difficult to isolate variables and explanations when in close proximity to the on-going research process and outcomes (see Sapsford and Abbott, 1992). However it is an approach to research that is often associated with a feminist or "human" philosophy to the research process.

Summary

It has been the aim of this chapter to introduce the concept of research and the philosophical approaches to research methods. The chapter commenced by reflecting upon the **nature of research** and the crucial process of setting the **research question(s)**. It was noted that research aims not to take for granted what many in health services do. It was also noted that research is an everyday experience. Many research projects are formulated in the questions we pose in talking to colleagues or privately reflecting on our professional practice.

Apart from the personal research project, undertaken as part of an educational course or for personal interest, **three main types of research** were identified, namely:

a.   the evaluation of new or existing practices;

b.   academic research creating or adding to a body of knowledge, and

c.   the evaluation of professional practice.

In any research project there are the confusion's and mistakes and this reality, whilst often denied in many texts, is explored in contributions to Part Two of this text.

The philosophical basis to research methods was identified as:

• qualitative, and

• quantitative.

In Table One these approaches were presented as a continuum with a range of methods for collecting data sitting at various points along this continuum. A **qualitative** approach proceeds from the principle of **induction**, namely in the exploration of issues and questions, patterns from which hypotheses may be generated. In a **quantitative** approach a hypothesis forms the provisional assumption and it is tested, and accepted or rejected as a consequence. Thus from the hypothesis testing a **deduction** is made.

Feminist approaches to research may incorporate both qualitative and quantitative methods but this approach is unique it its holistic approach to the totality of human experience, emotions and values in the research process. Implicit in this approach is the examination of power and authority as key components of ongoing oppression. **Action research** is an approach of feeding back results as an ongoing process; research in its activity is an on-going learning activity. This is an approach that is often combined with feminist principles.

References

Abbott P, Sapsford R (1992) *Research into Practice*. Open University Press, Buckingham

Daly J, McDonald I, Willis E (eds) (1992) *Researching Health Care. Designs, Dilemmas, Disciplines*. Routledge, London

Holland J, McKie L, Watson P (1994) *Promoting Women and Research*. British Sociological Association, Durham

Jones P (1993) *Studying Sociology*. Collins Educational, London

Najman J, Morrison J, Williams G, Andersen M (1992) Comparing Alternative Methodologies of Social Research. In: Daly, J *et al* (eds) *Researching Health Care*. Routledge, London, 138–157

Newell D (1992) Randomised Controlled Trials in Health Care Research. In: Daly *et al* (eds) *Researching Health Care*. Routledge, London, pp47–61

Oakley A (1993) *Essays on Women, Medicine and Health*. Edinburgh University Press, Edinburgh

Roberts H (ed) (1990) *Women's Health Counts*. Routledge, London

Roberts H (ed) (1992) *Women's Health Matters*. Routledge, London

Sapsford R, Abbott P (1992) *Research Methods for Nurses and the Caring Professions*. Open University Press, Buckingham

Stanley L, Wise S (1993) *Breaking Out Again*. Routledge, London

CHAPTER TWO
A RANGE of METHODS

Linda McKie

Introduction

In this chapter the range of methods available to the researcher are presented. Just as research questions differ so do potential research methods and those methods reflect the spectrum from inductive to deductive approaches. In this chapter a resumé of a number of methods is presented and further sources of information noted. The chapter commences with methods based upon the premise of inductive work, namely observation, discussion groups and interview techniques, moving to deductive methods, namely closed questionnaires and experimental design.

Observation

We have all acquired information and insight into a situation or event by observing who is present, what takes place, and how those present react. With a number of research methods, there is first hand contact with those participating in the research. For example, when booking appointments at a clinic the nurse meets women and observes their dress, their facial and body movements as well as hearing their words. From this we might judge who is happy, who is anxious or confused and respond accordingly.

But observation as a distinct research method draws a line between the casual observation, as suggested in the preceding paragraph, and observation as a means of acquiring data which permits a degree of interpretation. There exist a number of characteristics of observation as this distinct method, namely:

a. that it captures the social context in which a person or a groups' behaviour occurs;

b. that it captures significant events and, or activities that affect the social relations of the participants;

c. observation helps us to determine what constitutes reality from the standpoint of the world view, philosophy or outlook of the observed, and

d. it identifies regular events or activities, and recurrences in social life by comparing and contrasting data obtained in one study with those obtained in studies of other settings.

As Sapsford and Abbott (1992, p.6) note we are also active in the analysis of what we observe "seeing what we do as a result of the knowledge which we already have". Trying to make sense of a whole situation is not easy unless time is spent in immersing oneself in the situation. You need to achieve more than the description of a situation but to try and make sense of the "whole".

To achieve this level of understanding invariably requires the researcher to become part of a group or community. But that very process of becoming part of the "whole" alerts us to a major debate in this field or research, namely should the observer be a participant in the group or a non-participant observer? There are pluses and minuses with either approach. If you participate are you effecting the "naturalness" of the situation? How do you allow for the likely impact of your presence at, and input to, the group? Yet if you remain on the sidelines quietly observing will you fully comprehend and experience relationships between group members? Might also the notion of being "on the sidelines" enhance the group members sense of being scrutinised and thus further impact on group behaviour? In addition the amount of time that can be spent in observation can effect the nature of data. Is an event the researcher considers significant in fact a one off or a regular occurrence? Thus the simple task of using your vision and your presence to acquire information and insight is not without its drawbacks. And writing up the research data and experience can be a time consuming activity as this must both describe situations and present the analysis of data.

The observer must pay particular attention to the collection of data and subsequent analysis. Most observers maintain a diary, completed on a daily basis as well as immediately writing notes on any event or situation felt worthy of further analysis. Data might also be collected on tape, for example the taping or a group meeting, and also through visual representations, for example, photographs, written work or art work of the group. Thus the observer must be highly disciplined in note taking **and** ensure that all potential sources of written or visual data are recorded so the very wholeness of a social situation is available for analysis.

Analysis of observation data is both time consuming and potentially complex. The observer will first review data for commonalties. Where events occur on a regular basis or a certain form of words are used to describe an event the researcher will determine that the theme or words are a category. What is uncommon also becomes apparent and the unusual or irregular must be categorised. It is then possible to identify the frequency and distribution of phenomena.

Writing up an observation study requires an empathy for the reader who has not had the experiences of the researcher and for whom certain conclusions might appear unwarranted unless firmly located in an explanation of localities, individuals, relationships and events. The use of direct quotes with detailed description of individuals, localities and events can bring a social situation alive and give credence to your conclusions on a way of life or method of professional practice. Using this research method also gives a status to social experience which many researchers have denied.

When is observation appropriate?

There are a number of issues to consider when deciding upon the relevance of observation to a research project. These may be cited as:

a. the nature of the research question: certain research questions lend themselves more readily to observation as a method. For example examining life on a children's ward or researching the participation of the elderly in residential care would be better researched by observing the total social context. Are the children or elderly listened to? Are their views considered by some or all of the health care professionals in developing care? Clearly these questions involve a number of individuals from differing backgrounds coming together in a particular situation on a mutually relevant issue, namely the delivery of care. Situations in which vulnerable groups, or those less likely to be willing or able to talk to a researcher or complete a questionnaire, lend themselves more readily to observation. Similarly exploring professional practice or teamwork are also research issues more likely to be fully examined by observation. Who is speaking to whom? Communication, attitude and (in)actions may be observed in the context of the practice setting.

*b. the researcher's skills and personal characteristics:*the skills required to observe effectively rest upon the researchers appreciation of the impact of certain aggregate characteristics, namely, age, gender, race, dress and attitude. There are certain settings in which it may be difficult for certain researchers to be accepted and feel comfortable. For example a female researcher might feel uncomfortable observing in a male prison or a man might find observation problematic in an ante-natal clinic. It is important for the researcher to reflect upon the likely impact of themselves upon the research situation and to reflect critically upon this when writing up.

c. the characteristics of the observed: there are a number of settings in which observation may not be enough for full comprehension of a situation. For example doctors or solicitors may be working in complex situations with professional procedures that require further information to comprehend. Certain groups may also be disguising the reality of their situation while the researcher is present. For example, doctors have a public persona when working with patients which may make some proficient at concealing aspects of social situations and information. The very presence of a researcher may also make those present uneasy and wary of reacting in a natural manner. Attempting to determine the rules (the norms) and values in a situation can be difficult but observing everyday activities such as meal times and participating in social activities can assist in establishing the natural relationships in a given context. Finally economic concerns might also be factors in determining the response of respondents. In certain situations the presence of a researcher might inhibit the use of a service and the activities of patients or customers. As a consequence the researcher may not be welcome.

As noted earlier, the writing up of observation data can be time consuming; it takes time to adequately explain situations and present the evidence on which the analysis is based. Nevertheless the insight that can be gained from data collected by this method is invaluable in ensuring that the totality of a social situation can be identified and explored.

The discussion group

The discussion or focus group has become an increasingly popular method of data collection. As Morgan (1993) notes this is a method which few social scientists or other researchers had heard of as recently as five years ago. Yet it is a method that was developed in the 1930s by both psychologists and sociologists (e.g. Merton, et al, 1956). Its increasing popularity has often been linked to the assumption that it is an efficient and economical manner in which to gain responses from a number of respondents. But researcher beware! The discussion group can be time consuming to organise, complex to conduct and costly in both transcribing and analysis time. Nevertheless, it is a valuable component in the methods repertoire of any researcher, delivering a depth of data few methods can compete with. The discussion group is distinct from the group interview as it employs group interaction **as well as** group debate as research data (Kitzinger, 1993).

A basic description of the actual event of a discussion group appears uncontroversal. Discussions are organised to explore a set of topics or issues pre-determined by the research team (possibly, though not generally, in conjunction with respondents). Thus a key characteristic is the collective activity of considering the topics or, for example, a film or photograph. Discussions are taped with respondents asked to identify themselves on their initial contribution when speaking so that personal and interactive responses may be traced in any analysis. Personal and interactive discussions enhance the depth of data secured by encouraging people to say what they think, to illustrate how that thinking impacts on actions and to consider why they think as they do. People can relate views to actual events that they, their friends or relatives have experienced; they can relate folklore; they can place comments and stories in a longitudinal context, and most importantly they use there only words and interactive dialogue to illustrate their views and create a dialogue.

Setting up a discussion group can, as noted earlier, be time consuming. Making contact with pre-existing groups and asking the group to place your topic or activity on the agenda of a future meeting can be the most efficient method of getting discussion groups together. But a major drawback of this approach is that you meet only those who participate. Other methods of drawing people into groups can involve much leg and organisational work. Calling house to house or asking those who come along to a clinic to join a discussion group takes time. You also have to arrange a convenient and comfortable meeting place. All this generally costs money. While it is wise to keep numbers in groups of between 6 to 8 what do you do if no one or few turn up? Or if 12 or more arrive? With too few debate can be stifled and stilted. With too many it can be very difficult to pursue more than one theme, to keep all respondents interested and to identify on the tape who is actually speaking at any given point in time. It is, therefore, important to spend time ensuring you have a firm commitment from your respondents to attend. But who do you invite? The beauty of the discussion group is that you aim to elicit a range of variables within the context of group interaction. Thus your invitation list is likely to be both broad and related to the topic. For example, if your interest is in researching women's views of antenatal care you could invite a range of adult women — those who have given birth, those who have experienced any aspect of the service or those in fertile years and potentially likely to use the service — or you could focus upon women using a particular clinic who will have a recent experience of the service. This decision will be based upon the nature of the research question. A project which is concerned to fine tune current service might focus upon the views of current users. A project concerned with women's views of antenatal services and women's health more generally might consider a wider invitation list.

A member of the research team or the researcher must act as a facilitator ensuring that everyone in the group gets a chance to speak and that the group discusses topics of interest to themselves and the research questions. There is a fine dividing line between encouraging a group to explore an event and moving the conversation on by posing a further issue for group debate. Prior knowledge of group participants can be both an advantage and disadvantage as it can enhance initial debates but detract from actual explanations of events or issues; familiarity can lead to assumed knowledge. If this occurs the facilitator must ask questions. The facilitator may also need to ask questions or prompt discussion when group participants have little or no knowledge of each other. The ultimate goal is a flowing discussion as free from interruptions from the facilitator as possible, but as focused upon the research issues as can be reasonably achieved.

Setting objectives for a discussion group is a crucial step in clarifying the concepts or issues to be investigated. It is advisable to keep the topics or activities for consideration limited. Always consider an ice breaker topic to enhance the comfort and familiarity of those involved. Perhaps you could circulate the topics as a handout to everyone. Limit broad topics to between 4 and 6 issues. People get tired after an hour or so and their attention will drift off. So you must be focused. Pilot your topics list as you would with any method. And for the purposed of facilitation design a detailed checklist of items you would like the group to consider under the broad headings. For example you might consider communication with clinic staff as a broad topic of interest in the investigation of antenatal care. Within the debate on this topic you might want to check that the group considered the following questions:

- do you meet the same members of staff at each visit?

- do you consider that staff listen to your concerns, questions and views?

- is there any evidence or concerns expressed at the use of technical terms and medical jargon?

- how do women gain information? e.g. leaflets, classes or discussions

- what are respondents experiences of gaining further information on treatment or services?

- has anyone any experiences of making a complaint?

- any suggestions for changes in written or verbal communications?

So under a broad heading, which respondents are informed of, you would consider the points on the checklist ensuring that as many aspects of that topic as possible are considered.

Analysing data

Analysis of a taped discussion group first involves the transcribing of the data collected on tape. Be careful to decide beforehand how queues such as laughter, sarcasm, sorrow or concern might be coded as the manner in which a sentence is presented adds much to the meaning of words. Knodel (1993, p43) notes that "a considerable amount of subjective judgement is necessarily involved in ... interpretation and analysis". As noted above statements must be set in the wider context of group debate and the manner or tone of presentation. Transcripts of a one hour discussion can yield up to 30 pages of transcribed data for analysis.

There are two components in the analysis of discussion group data, namely mechanical and interpretative. In the first stage, mechanical, data is physically organised into meaningful but broad categories. This stage is often called "cutting and pasting". Data is physically moved across transcripts into broad categories for consideration. For example in considering data on antenatal care it may well be that certain issues such as location, staffing and waiting facilities are discussed across several groups. With the mechanical stage of analysis data on these three topics is physically brought together. At the interpretative stage the search is for patterns in the discussion within the broad categories. For example in discussing facilities at antenatal clinics it might become apparent that one clinic has poor facilities for children or staff are unsympathetic to long waiting times. However experiences at other clinics may differ and the impact of facilities on a woman's overall perceptions of care may also differ. It is useful at this stage to explore data categories with others in the research team and consider decisions as to the final categories identified as a group decision. Remember that while it is easy and very useful to identify similarities across groups it is also important to consider the dissimilarities or unique experiences presented.

There now exists two computer packages which assist with data analysis, namely, The Ethnograph and N.U.D.I.S.T. (Fielding and Lee, 1991) packages. Both require the typing in of data to a programmed PC and decisions as to the categories for analysis must still be made by the research team. But these programmes can cut down on the mass of paper that tends to go with the cut and paste method by typing out only those quotes relevant to a pre-determined category. However it is advisable that those new to interpretative data analysis commence with the cut and paste method as the sheer physical proximity to the data can assist in considering categories for the allocation of data.

Having decided upon your categories, a grid should then be produced with categories on one axis and identifiers for a discussion group on the other. Cells would contain a brief summary of the content of data allocated to that cell. Develop your own code system as such an overview cannot physically contain all relevant data. A numbering system for quotes of a particular type or key words might be employed. This process should be conducted for both each group and for a total overview, a grid produced for all groups together. Again a team approach to this process is imperative as it enhances reliability and the quality of data analysis.

Writing up discussion group data posses similar issues to that of observation data. The characteristics of group members must be described and it is useful to consider collecting brief socio-economic data from respondents. Don't forget that the location and nature of accommodation can impact upon the discussion. One person might dominate or certain people not participate. You need to alert the reader to the decision processes in interpreting data and reflect on this when deciding upon categories. Actual quotes bring categories to life for the reader, and it is important to point out both similarities and dissimilarities across groups.

When is the discussion group an appropriate method?

Morgan and Kruger (1993, pp19) suggest a number of advantages in this method, namely:

a. it is a useful method when a power differential exists between participants and decision makers as it allows peers to express their opinions as a group hopefully ensuring a level of security and mutual support;

b. likewise it is a useful method when there is a gap between professionals and their target audiences, not only because of power and information differentials but also as it provides a useful forum for exploring how groups think and express views on a topic;

c. when considering complex behaviours or motivations this method can begin the process of understanding the how and the why when exploring personal, intimate or controversial issues, e.g., views on HIV/AIDS;

d. it is a method which allows researchers to learn what is known about a topic through the group exploration of an item or issue, and

e. it is a method with a "unique niche for obtaining information as tensions between opposing parties begin to rise" (Morgan and Krueger, *ibid*). In fact, the process of conducting a discussion group can demonstrate and create a trust and manner of working which can set the foundations for future work amongst a range of people.

In addition, Kitzinger (1993) suggests that it is a method that is essential to any understanding of attitudes and can, in its conduct, help to construct beliefs and attitudes. As a consequence, it is a useful method of both challenging and creating views amongst group members.

The interview

The interview can be conducted on either a one-to-one or a group basis. This method differs from the discussion group in that questions are posed by the researcher. The questions may be open ended (seeking speculation) or closed (requiring short information based answers).

This method is a good means of finding out what people think on an issue. Data may also be derived from the verbal interaction between the researcher and respondent(s). There are a number of characteristic features of the interview, namely:

a. it is an act of verbal communication for the purpose of eliciting information (Denzin, 1970). It may be conducted in person or over the phone;

b. in the conduct of the interview both parties behave as though they are of equal status - whether this is actually the case - for the duration of the interview;

c. those involved demonstrate a uniformity in behaviour. For example, as appropriate either may listen when a question is asked or an answer given. This uniformity gives a stability and security to the event which enhances equality, the potential comfort of those involved and, hopefully, the quality of data;

d. information is recorded by the researcher either on tape or through note taking (although it should be noted that note taking can detract from eye to eye conduct and inhibit the flow of the verbal communication);

e. it is a transitory relationship; it is, generally, a new experience for those involved, and

f. it allows for the collection of data in settings convenient to respondents. For example interviewing the nurse during a surgery or clinic time is unlikely to be convenient for either the researcher or respondent, nor is it likely to enhance the quality of data.

The interview method allows for a variability of settings and times to enhance mutual understanding of both questions and answers. While there is often a format of questions it is a method which allows for spontaneity. It is a method that is also very productive with those likely to find a questionnaire difficult to read or complete, e.g. the young, the elderly, the mentally ill or mentally handicapped. It is useful in situations where the busy worker or mum can have their views written down by the researchert. And many researchers now conduct a series of interviews as a precursor to writing a questionnaire as it elicits issues and language of relevance to further respondents.

The interview enhances exploration of a topic between respondent and researcher but there exist a number of factors which affect the use of the interview as a method. These factors include:

a. the objective and subjective qualities of the interviewer. Objective qualities include the appropriateness of the interviewers age, gender, socio-economic class, dress and accent. Subjective factors to consider include the ability of the researcher to maintain a flow in the interview discussion especially if it is a group interview, and to draw together scattered and disjointed pieces of information, and

b. the qualities of the respondent(s). These may be cited as interest, motivation, abilities to respond and potential conflict in responding to a pre-determined series of questions. As with any method, respondents interest and motivation may vary; busy people may be best interviewed over the phone. You may have refusals as people may not perceive the relevance of the research to themselves and others may agree, reluctantly, and demonstrate that reluctance in their answers. Language difficulties, and hearing and sight disabilities may make the conduct of the interview more complex and possibly suggest a further method as more appropriate, e.g. observation. In addition, the status and/or views of a respondent may result in conflict over the shaping of the interview and wording of the questions. For example a doctor might query why you are asking particular questions and this dialogue may well divert you from the pre-designed conduct of the interview.

Types of interviews: structured and unstructured

There are two commonly cited types of interviews which form a continuum ranging from the structured to the unstructured interview. Ay one end of this continuum lies the structured interview in which questions are pre-set, regulated and the researcher moves through the questions in the pre-determined order. At the other end of the continuum lies the unstructured interview in which the questions form a guide to the discussion and the interviewer follows the flow of the conservation adding questions as appropriate. The reality for the researcher is that the interview will probably demonstrate aspects of both types and dependent upon the topic and situation the type of interview will fall somewhere on the continuum between structured and unstructured interviews.

Structured interviews have a quality of "sameness" in their conduct which makes comparability possible. There also exist a number of pluses and minuses with this type of interview, namely:

a.   recording costs may be less and coding more efficient as data will usually follow pre-determined lines;

b.   there will be less tendency for data to move from the dominant topic of the research;

c. however this very quality of the structured interview process may result in a loss of spontaneity and thus loss of relevant data, and

d. the potential for exploring points raised by respondents is limited.

By contrast unstructured interviews make a positive use of spontaneity as a means of acquiring data. The interview context is as free of regulation and conscious constraint as possible. There exist a number of advantages and disadvantages with this type of interview. These may be summarised as follows:

a. apart from the spontaneity element there is also the centrality of the interviewees responses to the process which results in less researcher bias and a potentially more comfortable and pleasing experience to the interviewee;

b. in addition a key advantage is the exploration of issues in an unrestricted manner thus further illuminating an issue or topic, and

c. the disadvantages are threefold;

   • the comparability of data may be problematic;

   • interviews may generate unique data;

   • the classification of responses may be time consuming, and

   • the views of the respondent(s) may be irrelevant to the research topic.

Clearly the research question to be explored will indicate which type of interview to adopt. However the interview as a method, regardless of type, ensures that information can be obtained is a reasonable efficient manner, from relevant respondents and allows a flexibility in its organisation. Interviewer and interviewee bias remain as potential problems as does the time involved in the conduct of interviews and analysis of data. Ultimately the interview capitalises on the most natural form of social communication, the conversation.

One final point for the reader; data analysis follows the same lines as the analysis of the discussion group data. Please refer to the preceding section of this chapter for an outline of a potential process for analysis.

The Questionnaire

The questionnaire continues to be a very popular method of data collection. The functions of the questionnaire are to provide:

a. individual and group characteristics such as gender, age, years of full time or part time education, current and previous occupation, income, political and religious affiliation, membership of groups etc;

b. frequencies, by collating numbers and attributing data to categories such as gender, age bands, occupational types, and

c. data for other statistical tests such as cross tabulations which measure the strength of a relationship between two or more variables (Vogt, 1993).

The questionnaire allows for the measurement of individual or group variables such as how many women attended a clinic on a particular day; who saw which consultant or nurse, and how long did anyone wait to be seen? Through statistical tests it allows for the testing of the strength of a relationship between variables, for example, whether women who attended on any particular day had to wait for more than 30 minutes, thus assessing the relationship, if any, between clinic days starting and waiting times. However the questionnaire is not a method best disposed to obtaining views of respondents nor establishing the wider context of those views. This results from the composition of questions written by the researcher and research team, These questions reflect the decisions made by the researcher as to what to incorporate and how to word the questions. In addition questionnaires often provide respondents with a choice of answers, and these choices may restrict responses and reflect the categories designed by the research team. The potential problems with the questionnaire are related to the pre-determination of questions and answers.

Types of questions and questionnaire composition

There exist two types of questions; namely, fixed response or closed questions and open questions:

a. in fixed response or closed questions the respondent is asked to check a range of responses and select the one they consider most appropriate. This is a quick and easy method of collecting data which promotes completion rates. A major problem is that none of the responses may be appropriate to a respondent and the 'catch-all' category "other" is noted giving the research little insight into the respondent's views or characteristics, and

b. open questions require replies worded by respondents and this allows respondents to elaborate on their opinions and attitudes. This is a more time-consuming method of collecting data through questionnaires and it requires a level of verbal and possibly written skills that cannot be assumed from all respondents. It may also be difficult for interviewers, in administering a questionnaire, to note responses verbatim.

Many questionnaires combine both fixed response and open questions, using fixed response questions to acquire descriptive information such as age, gender, occupation and open questions to obtain views and attitudes.

Analysis of question types does differ. With fixed response questions analysis commences with the attribution of a pre-set code to each specific response. With the category "other" and open questions the research team must decide upon categories of responses (as with discussion group and interview data) and attribute a code to the determined categories. This can result in a large number of categories, and thus codes, making the use of certain statistical testing difficult. However the calculation of frequencies can still be undertaken.

Constructing and administering the questionnaire

It is extremely important to pilot any questionnaire prior to final administration to respondents. At the initial composition stage there are a number of issues to consider:

a. selecting the topics for questions; careful research is required to ascertain any previous questionnaires constructed on your research area. This assists in alerting you to topic areas for questions as does a review of research literature in the area. Many researchers choose to run one or two discussion groups prior to writing their questionnaire. This has a number of benefits such as highlighting the relevant issues to potential respondents and ensuring that the words and phrases employed by a certain population are used in any questionnaire thus enhancing respondent comprehension, the number and quality of responses;

b. the wording of questions; as noted above the wording must reflect the language commonly employed by respondent groups. For example teenagers will employ slang language and discussions on sex and health amongst a range of groups commonly employ euphemisms;

c. the sequence of a series of questions must be carefully thought through and tested at a piloting stage. What are the functions of particular questions? For example, is description of the respondents or measurement of events required? Are fixed response or open questions required? Fixed response questions are easy to complete and are a good introduction to the exercise for questionnaire respondents. Open questions requiring reflection and greater time to complete might be better placed at the end of a section or the questionnaire, and

d.   the noting of non-respondents and reasons for declining to complete a questionnaire should be undertaken. At the piloting stage such responses might provide a useful insight into any potential controversies or problems. Of course it must be remembered that any respondent has the right to refuse participation in research and this decision should be respected.

The administration of any questionnaire can be by post — for self-completion; face to face with an interviewer or researcher — for self-completion with guidance, or face to face — for completion by an interviewer noting responses. Administrating a questionnaire by post invariably requires the sending out of a reminder, after a suitable time period, to enhance the response rate. The administration of a questionnaire by an interviewer does tend to result in less refusals and a greater quality of answers but it is time consuming and demanding of resources. Research budgets and the timetable for the research programme are invariably the determinants of which approach to the administration of the questionnaire is adopted.

Analysis

The coding of questionnaires must be considered at the design stage of the questionnaire. With fixed response questions each answer is number and the appropriate number placed in a coding box relevant to the question. Responses to open questions are categorised after questionnaire completion and coded accordingly. Apart from the calculation of frequencies, i.e. the quantification of the number giving a particular response to a question which is calculated as a percentage figure, there exists a range of statistical tests which may be employed to examine and test the strength of variables. The range and choice of statistical tests is the subject of a number of text books which the reader should consider at the design stage of any project employing a questionnaire (see Gilbert, 1992; Floyd and Fowler, 1993; Vogt, 1993).

The Controlled Trial

This is a method most commonly associated with clinical research. The control trial aims to:

a. measure change in a group who have received a treatment or intervention, and

b. establish that any measurable change has occurred as a consequence of the treatment or intervention.

To establish that change has in fact resulted from the intervention, respondents are allocated on a random basis to a treatment group and to a group which will not receive treatment known as the control group. A comparison of appropriate measurements can then be made at the end of the intervention to establish whether:

a. definable and quantifiable change has taken place amongst respondents in the treatment group, and

b. that any change has resulted from the treatment or intervention.

However both groups should receive as similar an experience as possible. For example in a drug trial one group will receive the drug the other a placebo. In addition it is necessary to match the membership of the groups, e.g., participants could be matched for age, gender, occupation and medical condition. This takes time but is an invaluable part of the experimental process. It is, however, the researcher who matches and allocates participants and bias may result. In addition the knowledge by respondents that they are receiving a new treatment may in itself produce change resultant from that knowledge rather than from the treatment. This is commonly known as the "Hawthorne Effect" (named after the location of a series of trials in the 1920s when this effect was noted). To avoid the "Hawthorne Effect" the double blind technique is employed and neither group members are actually made aware whether they are, for example, receiving the new drug or the placebo (see Lewis-Beck, 1993).

Not surprisingly the randomised control trial which employs the double blind technique has been criticised as unethical for it conceals knowledge from the patient and restricts access to a treatment which may be of benefit to the patient. In addressing some of these criticisms researchers have developed a further approach known as the partially randomised control trial (Henshaw *et al*, 1993). In this approach patients are fully informed of the available treatments and asked to decide whether they wish to join the project and, if so, do they wish to join the intervention or control group. If patients express no preference then they are randomly allocated to a group. This method is best employed in situations where treatment types are being compared in situation where treatment should take place, for example two types of surgical interventions both aiming to relieve a particular medical or physical condition. Matching in this method can become highly problematic and it is best employed in situations where the outcome will be some form of intervention and the views and preferences of patients on the available treatments may determine future practices.

There are no practical examples of the control trial in this text. It is a method largely employed for clinical research purposes and there are examples in a number of texts, further exploring the control trial method (see Lewis-Beck, 1993; Sapsford and Abbott, 1992; Abbott and Sapsford, 1992).

Sampling

There exist a number of methods of selecting a sample of respondents, namely:

- the probability sample

- the stratified random sample

- the simple random sample

- the systematic random sample or quota sample

- the snowball technique

The conclusions that may be drawn from a study are contingent upon the nature of the sample. It is, therefore, extremely important that any researcher considers the various possibilities of sample selection and in reporting the research notes the approach adopted giving the advantages and disadvantages of the selected approach.

Probability and non probability sampling

The starting point for sampling is the census or other indexes of populations such as the community health index in Scotland. The census, in the UK conducted every ten years, is a tabulation of all persons in the population. The probability sample is a portion of that population made up of persons who all have an equal choice of being drawn into the sample. The key advantage with this approach is that the concept of equal chance for selection restricts researcher bias.

In a non probability sample a set of people are chosen for their possession of certain characteristics or for the convenience of the researcher working with time and resource constraints. With the stratified random sample a weighting is given to particular sub groups of the total population so that samples with specific characteristics are selected. For example an equal number of old and young. In addition the population may be stratified, say according to age or gender. If your research is concerned with the views of an equal number of young men and women participating in 16 plus sex education, the strata would be gender, age and educational status. In the simple random sample selections are based upon a lottery, say the 1st and every third person in a census list. In the quota sample the selection is based upon a lottery but the list from which people are drawn is already comprised of those possessing characteristics central to the research question (see Gilbert, 1992: Sapsford and Abbott, 1992).

Triangulating data

Many research projects now combine a range of methods. In the chapters by Gregory and McKie, and Posner a multi-method approach was taken to ensure that various dimensions of a service were chartered, for example both the characteristics of service users and the views of service users. Interviews and discussion groups are often employed to illuminate topics for questionnaires and the wording of specific questions. Triangulating data from multiple sources can be used "to corroborate, elaborate, or illuminate the research in question" (Marshall and Rossman, 1989, p146). The process of triangulation generally involves the use of a range of research methods enhancing a study's generalisability by examining the same research question from several perspectives.

Summary

In this chapter a number of methods were outlined ranging along the qualitative, qualitative continuum from observation to the randomised control trial. The methods outlined were:

- observation
- discussion groups
- interviews
- questionnaires
- the controlled trial.

Consideration was given to sampling as a critical aspect of research design and any assessment in the reliability of a project. Multi-method projects are increasingly evident. In these projects a number of methods are combined and these methods may reflect the qualitative and quantitative approaches. The collection of data from several triangulation perspectives, can be used to ascertain reliability and validity.

One final suggestion. It does pay to be honest in reporting the advantages and disadvantages of the chosen method or methods. There are draw backs with every method and recognising these allows the reader to assess the reliability of the research. Just because you do not outline the disadvantages of your chosen approach does not mean that the reader will be any less aware of the draw backs in the methods applied. Reflection upon the methods applied allows you to evaluate the outcomes of your project and build upon this experience for future research work.

References

*****BMJ article on partially randomised control trial******

Abbott P, Sapsford R (1992) *Research into Practice: a Reader for Nurses and the Caring Professions.* Open University Press, Buckingham

Fielding N, Lee R (1991) *Using Computers in Qualitative Research* Sage, London

Floyd J, Fowler Jr (1993) *Survey Research Methods* Sage, London

Gilbert N (1992) *Researching Social Life.* Sage, London

Henshaw R, Naji S, Russell I, Templeton A (1993) Comparison of medical abortion with surgical vacuum aspiration: Women's preferences and acceptability of treatment. *Br Med J* 307: 714–7

Kitzinger J (1993) The Methodology of Focus Groups: the Importance of Interaction Between Research Participants. *Sociol Health Illness* 161: 103–121

Knodel J (1993) The Design and Analysis of Focus Group Studies: A Practical Approach. In: Morgan, D (ed) *Successful Focus Groups*. Sage, London: 35–50

Lewis-Beck M (ed) (1993) *Experimental Design and Methods*. Sage, London

Merton R *et al* (1956) *The Focused Interview: A Report of the Bureau of Applied Social Research*. Columbia University, New York

Morgan D (ed) (1993) *Successful Focus Groups*. Sage, London

Morgan D, Kruger R (1993) When to Use Focus Groups and Why, In: Morgan D (ed) *Successful Focus Groups*. Sage, London: 19

Sapsford R, Abbott P (1992) *Research Methods for Nurses and the Caring Professions*. Open University Press, Buckingham

Vogt P (1993) *Dictionary of Statistics and Methodology. A Non-Technical Guide for the Social Scientist* Sage, London

CHAPTER THREE
WOMEN'S EXPERIENCES of INFERTILITY: SOME SHARED ENCOUNTERS

Jane Wills

Abstract

This study explores women's experiences of infertility and their different perceptions of infertility as a medical, social and psycho-social issue. A central concern was to make infertility more visible and show how a narrow medical view in relation to treatment or services ignores the powerful feelings and implications for the mind and social relationships. The methodology is based on the concept of a shared encounter between researcher and researched and the influences shaping this approach are described based on personal experience and a critique of traditional forms of inquiry.

Infertility has tended to be regarded narrowly as a medical issue requiring diagnosis, treatment and, hopefully, a 'cure' involving pregnancy. The focus is on the body's reproductive capacity: the implications for the mind and on social relationships are largely ignored. In the field of health education, a woman's right to choose not to have children (through the availability of contraception and abortion) has assumed far greater importance than the fight to ensure that they can.

This study was undertaken as part of a higher degree in Health Education in 1989 (Wills 1992). Its purpose was to capture and describe women's unique experience of infertility as part of her whole life. It explores different perceptions of infertility - as a medical, social and psycho-social issue - by exploring with a small group of women their experiences of infertility. It sought to explore a role for health education in self-empowerment, in encouraging an awareness of choice and providing knowledge and opportunities for women to explore and understand their own bodies.

Theoretical context

The importance of undertaking personally important research has been stressed by Rowan and Reason in their critique of scientific research (Rowan and Reason, 1981). The basic premise of this New Paradigm research is that research should be with and for (not on) people. It sets aside the scientific notion of objectivity and that researchers should seek to eliminate all forms of bias and value judgement. No research is value-free. All researchers have their own personal and historical reasons for doing that research, in that way and at that particular time. My interest and reasons for choosing to explore the area of infertility were influenced by my own experience of infertility investigations over several years. I had become actively involved in achieving my goal of a child: talking, joining organisations and a support group, seeking out information, reading avidly, trying various self-help remedies and pursuing medical investigations. Although I discovered I was by no means alone in my inability to have a child, infertility seemed an `invisible subject'. It is an immensely powerful experience and I wanted to find some way of giving voice to these feelings, not what caused it, how it could be defined or how it could be changed, but what it means in the context of people's lives. Far from regarding my experience as a hindrance or skew on research in this area, I wished to adopt a methodology that would allow a pooling of insights and a sharing of experience. The relationship between researcher and researched to become one of equality and mutual inquiry, shifting power from the researcher who is giving of herself.

Medicine has had a controlling role in the definition and management of infertility. The underlying assumption of reproductive medicine is that fertility is a `fact' of nature and thus there is an objective criterion for the definition of infertility:

A woman is considered infertile if she has been continuously exposed to the risk of pregnancy for two years and has not conceived (Diczafalusy, 1985).

The medical model thus looks to the reproductive system to diagnose the condition and the cure. The language of infertility refers to `mechanical problems' such as tubal blockages which the doctor seeks to repair. There is even a diagnostic category of `unexplained infertility'. In other words, medicine has yet to uncover the cause. The orientation is then to more medicine: genetic screening; investigations of reproductive function; new techniques such as *in-vitro* fertilisation (IVF), gamete intra-fallopian transfer (GIFT), embryo transfer. Parsons saw this as part of the social control function of medicine (Parsons, 1951). Once infertility is a recognised condition, women must want to leave that role and get well and are thus obliged to seek and comply with medical advice. Thus, medicine attempts to reintegrate the deviant or unfit through its curative aspects but also acts as an agency of socialisation by ensuring the possibility of motherhood. This study sought to uncover whether, and in what ways, women who are well but encouraged to see themselves as abnormal, do perceive and explain their infertility as a medical issue.

This study was undertaken as part of a higher degree in Health Education which influenced its direction. Health education has long been dominated by a preventive approach. Its role in so far as it has taken up infertility, has been to highlight those aspects of lifestyle which may cause fertility problems, including sexually transmitted diseases, drinking, smoking, nutrition and, to a lesser extent, environmental hazards. The emphasis has been on information-giving with the intention of bringing about behaviour change. One purpose of this study was then to explore with women, the kinds of support they would expect and hope for from Health Education.

There is a developed feminist position which argues that infertility should be seen in the context of systematic oppression in society (Corea, 1985; Arditti, 1984). That oppression is manifested in the dominance of medicine and patriarchal and pronatal conditioning which socialises women into an expectation of motherhood. Whilst reproductive information and medicine offer women increased choices, such choices are determined by the social structure which creates the needs which lead to the desire for choice — the need to be a mother, the need to have a small family, the need for perfect children (Arditti, 1984). This study sought to explore with women their views on motherhood and how expectations of motherhood and family had shaped their experiences.

Infertility is not a prominent issue in health debates on the Right or Left (Berer, 1985). A campaign against infertility research involving embryos and new techniques has been led by religious groups and the Right. The only argument from the Left has been that infertility should be part of a wider struggle to ensure more responsive and available services for women in the NHS. In the light of the emphasis on consumerism and client needs in a changing National Health Service, this study explored how women regard their reproductive choices.

Methodology

Reason and Hawkins (1988) suggest there are two paths of inquiry in any study — explanation and expression. Explanation is the model of scientific inquiry into the material world, expression is the model of understanding the meaning of the social or mental world; and the two are complementary poles of a dialectic. Explanation without understanding is sterile; expression without explanation is insight without rigour or method. This study attempts a combination of understanding with rigour. It departs from conventional social research in several key areas.

Firstly, social research pursues a pseudo-scientific model as is evidenced by the traditional concern for hypothesis-making, falsification, objectivity and numbers. Yet science is but one form of knowledge, or way of viewing the world, and its basic precepts stem from a socially acquired corpus of knowledge (Chalmers, 1982). Scientific study has been associated with a masculine view of the world; as a form of alienated activity which is more concerned with controlling knowledge than understanding (Keller, 1983). Subjective knowledge, understanding and experience is not valued. As Hochschild (1975) observes, there is no subject area within social science devoted to the study of feelings and emotions, not she argues because of a lack of data or its unsociological character but because the cognitive, intellectual and rational dimensions of experience are seen as superior to the emotional or sentimental. The focus of this study was to acknowledge a holistic view of health and explore affective areas of experience.

Secondly, crucial to scientific method is the notion of objectivity and any form of bias must be eliminated. Social scientists studying other human beings can never be truly objective. Their own social concepts and values inevitably underpin every stage of the study. However, it is possible to critically reflect on one's own involvement and make explicit one's ideology (Mannheim, 1936). Inherent in value-free research is the treatment of people as research objects. The researcher is to stand back from the study and see it dispassionately and objectively. Implicitly, the researcher is powerful,determining the focus and being able to use their training and skill to analyse others' lives even more than those who actually live them. This study replaces such attempts at neutrality with what Klein (1983) has called 'conscious partiality' — identification with the so-called 'objects' of the study, such that they become subjects. This is different from simple empathy or subjective experience. The relationship allows the researcher to share her experiences as a woman and as a researcher with the participant.

Thirdly, conventional research suggests that any study requires an orienting theory to indicate which phenomena are important to study and how to frame the research question. All research is influenced by its context be it the source of funding or, as in this case, the nature of the degree for which it was submitted. It was, therefore, necessary for this study to draw out some implications for health education. Beyond that, it seemed important that subjects should speak for themselves and meaning should emerge from a negotiated interpretation of the data (Glaser and Strauss, 1969). Thus, interviews were totally unfocussed and the themes were chosen by the subjects and no assumptions were made about what was or was not important.

Participatory research suggests that subjects should be co-respondents in the identification of priorities and the collection and interpretation of information. In this study, the degree of control exercised by subjects was not as extensive as I would have wished. Subjects were able to determine the direction of interviews and to this extent controlled their own narrative. They reflected on the interview process and each woman reviewed the presentation of her material. However, research that is funded or carried out for vocational purposes is not shared and the intention and rationale remains that of the researcher.

Fourthly, the aim of scientific inquiry is to arrive at generalisable results which can then explain behaviours. It rejects the particular as essentially subjective and not 'scientific'. This study was concerned to capture and describe each woman's unique experience. It was not the intention to formulate a general view of infertility. It presents the experience of seven women. Is seven too few for 'reasonable' statements to be made? When the same themes, issues and topics emerge from those interviewed, is it possible to draw out some generalisations? Like most qualitative researchers, I felt under pressure to produce more data even though the purpose of the study was to prioritise meaning and values. Whilst this was an active theoretical choice, methodology is also dictated by practical concerns of time and funding. Qualitative investigations of this kind generate enormous amounts of data and therefore, its numbers must be limited.

The process of the research

The purpose of this research was to gain understanding of the experience of infertility. As mutuality and trust are crucial components of qualitative research, only women were part of this study. Oakley (1981) and Finch (1984) have suggested that women are able to appeal to what is common to women and their life experience and thus build deeper and more trusting relationships.

Women are more used than men to accepting intrusions through questioning into the more private parts of their lives......I have often been aware of an identification, as women interviewees have begun to talk about key areas of their lives in ways which denote a high level of trust in me, and indicate that they expect me to understand what they mean simply because I am another woman (Finch, 1984).

A second principle of the methodology was the sharing of experience. This would only be possible with another woman who was experiencing infertility. A more pragmatic reason for not including men in the study was due to the difficulties of gaining access. Numerous studies have highlighted the difficulties men have in talking about infertility, reflecting a general difficulty in expressing emotions but also the associations made between infertility and virility which makes men especially vulnerable (Pfeffer and Woollett, 1983; Houghton and Houghton, 1984; Stanway, 1980).

As I could only process a small number of interviews as part of this unfunded study undertaken at the same time as full-time work, I decided to use a snowball or opportunity sample. This method of selection recruits subjects on the basis of personal introduction (networking). Through my own efforts to be more open and visible about my infertility, I had met many others who were involuntarily childless. A group of seven women were chosen who were either known to me personally, introduced by a friend or part of an infertility support group I attended. This method of recruitment had the added advantage of familiarity and informality but it by no means assured rapport or sharing.

In all instances, I contacted the women by telephone explaining that I was doing a research study on women's experience of infertility. I explained that my interest arose from my own years of infertility investigations. I wanted to indicate at the outset that the experience was a shared one and that I was no longer childless. For some women in certain stages of living with infertility, contact with pregnant women or mothers can be painful. I asked the women if they would be willing to share their experience.

Opportunity samples can make no claims to being representative and this would have been difficult due to the lack of epidemiological data on who is affected by infertility and whether it is socially or economically distributed (Warnock, 1985). The seven women who were interviewed were all in their thirties; living in London; college-educated and had long histories of full-time employment. All were owner-occupiers and owned a car. Six of the women were white. All were living in heterosexual relationships. Since my concern was to give a voice to each person's experience, I was not concerned about typical qualities. A more central issue was what criterion of infertility should be used. Whether, for example, there should be a specific period of trying to conceive or only women undergoing investigations. What seemed more important than any such objective criteria was a woman's own definition and whether she regarded herself as infertile or involuntarily childless - temporarily or not. All women were, in fact, undergoing investigations and the length of time trying to conceive ranged from eighteen months to five years.

It was decided that in-depth interviews would be the most appropriate method to enable women to express the experience of infertility. There are many different ways of interviewing.

Traditional technique suggests that the researcher has a prepared list of focused questions both to establish a structure and for ease of subsequent analysis but also to maintain distance from the researched. These interviews would have two key elements — they would give as much control as possible to the subjects and they were to be **shared** encounters. There was no schedule of questions and no overall direction and as much time as the subject desired. The interview started with an explanation of its purpose and a guarantee of anonymity and control over the written material. I then indicated to the women that there would be no specific questions and I hoped we would be able to pool our experiences, feelings and understanding. I asked the women `tell me the story of your infertility'. This open invitation produced long factual accounts about how long they had been trying to get pregnant and their medical investigations. Occasionally, I would ask a simple question to invite an account of feelings: 'How did that make you feel?' Questions were, however, limited and typically, I used techniques such as feedback and reflection derived from non-directive counselling. My own involvement was to echo the subject's experience, either of my own accord but more usually I was asked if I had found a similar experience. Frequently, I was asked for factual information on infertility investigations. Oakley, in her study on maternity, also noted this process whereby the researcher becomes a source of information for the researched. She suggests that women researching women may well thus become involved in the interview process and it is indicative of the greater equality of the relationship (Oakley, 1981). The interviews took from one to five hours, sometimes spanning whole evenings. They were taped and transcribed and subjects were able to make any changes and reflect on what they had got out of the encounter.

The presentation of a qualitative study confronts the researcher with an immediate problem of how to handle the mass of data generated by depth interviews. Transcribing taped interviews takes, on average, four times as long as the interview itself. Thus, whilst it is important for subjects to speak for themselves, inevitably the presentation of the study involves selection and editing of material.

A narrative approach to the presentation of data stresses the importance of the story and the emphasis is on analysing the content in its original form. This includes several readings of the transcripts, immersing oneself in what is said, both text and sub-text. These stories are richly embedded and anecdotes contain many references to themes and aspects of health and infertility. Since there were no prior questions and the interviews range and return over several areas, it is important not to pluck out sections of narrative to support preconceived notions. In the presentation, broad themes have been identified which were signalled by subjects as important or which recurred in all the accounts.

A true account of each encounter would also involve more than a verbal transcript which cannot begin to convey the atmosphere and flow which makes each interview unique. Massarik (1981) has described the interview result as:

> *a document revelatory of both interviewer and interviewee, chronicling the process and content of their evolving exploration.*

It was also important as part of the methodological enquiry to explore how far these encounters were shared and the levels of control and influence. The original presentation of this study thus incorporated a phenomenological map which drew from common-sense categories of interaction (Wills, 1989). This showed for each encounter, the order in which themes emerged; the researcher's contributions; the extent of responses; the level of interest and energy; where control was taken by the subject and where by myself; non-verbal contributions and negative emotional spaces.

Although I was looking for some way of providing a replica of each encounter, limitations of time and space meant reducing the material to a manageable form. In so doing, I am aware I am robbing the individual encounter of its wholeness and doing only limited justice to the richness and complexity of any interaction.

Discussion of findings

Several broad themes emerged from this study relating to women's perceptions of infertility as a medical issue. These have been categorised as: the body as a machine, the body under siege and the body as a whole using some of the categories adopted by Stainton Rogers to explore perceptions of health and illness (Stainton Rogers, 1991). Consideration is also given to infertility as a social issue and the ways in which women had come to want children and how they now saw themselves when childless. Infertility is an immensely powerful experience likened to personal crisis. The psycho-social experience is explored through women's accounts of themselves under pressure.

The body as a machine

All the women in this study had chosen to pursue medical investigations and believed that doctors would find an answer for them. The acceptance that medicine will define and control the experience of infertility even extended to those women who rejected the label of 'infertile' but nevertheless had sought medical help for reassurance.

> "I think it's just to exclude your worst fear which is 'you've got this terrible problem and you'll never be able to'. It's really to exclude things, to reassure me that if we keep on trying, it will happen naturally. I think it's linked to wanting to know in advance, the points, to exclude certain points when you know there may be problems [Karen]."

The medical pathologising of reproduction encompasses infertility as well as childbirth and women become passive objects of clinical attention. Medicine is the main source of constructs and integral to the way most women perceive their childlessness. All the women in this study saw themselves as 'having something wrong' and saw having a baby as their sole goal. They had come to depend on the doctor to determine which investigations to carry out, to provide explanations. and to determine their eligibility for specialised treatments.

Most women welcomed the choices offered by new reproductive technologies, but each had her own limits to how far she would take her desire for a child. For some, a genetic link was important which excluded donor insemination and adoption; others felt the stress of in vitro fertilisation (IVF) programmes and adoption procedures to be too great and some regarded IVF as meddling with a natural process.

The body under siege

Most women in accepting a label of 'infertile' had come to rely on medical treatment yet most lacked information about treatment procedures, its risks and possible outcomes. The wanted to be good patients and so co-operated in treatments without knowing why:

"I don't know why they are doing the tests. It's always that they are in control and so I feel I have to do as I'm told. I used to ring days on my temperature chart when we were supposed to have had intercourse. I think I thought otherwise I would be wasting their time [Mary]

They're only concerned what's the next treatment they're going to give you. Even 'X' who's a good doctor, just didn't know what to say and so we've got put on an IVF programme. I suppose because you're so desperate and because it's the only thing that's offering anything, you accept that stuff. In terms of high technology... you don't have a choice... well you do have a choice — to remain childless [Jean]

Several women, acutely aware of their loss of control over their bodies and the apparent arbitrariness of infertility, stressed feelings of guilt and blame. They searched for things in their past with which to blame themselves — perhaps because they put off getting pregnant, because of sexual infections, because they smoke:

> *I do worry whether I am too uptight but then I become more uptight and when I was in my early twenties and I had quite a log of sexual relationships and I think I had NSU (Non Specific Uretheritis) one time and whether that had something to do with it [Jean]*

The body as a whole

Two women drew upon religion in their accounts of infertility. Margaret, who described herself as a practising Catholic, regarded God and prayer as the major sources of healing although she was able to interweave this with an acceptance of medicine:

> *"God will look after me. If I do everything I possibly can and trust in him, whatever will be and if I have faith it will be all right". [Margaret]*

Mary was able to explore her feeling that infertility was a form of punishment:

> *"There's a bit of me that thinks 'It serves me right' because, you should have done it younger, stayed married...like a punishment from some power" [Mary]*

The tremendous well of recovery in each person characterised Karen's account:

> *"I don't think one should think about it too much. I don't want negative feelings to take over my life. If I can respect myself for all the ways I am other things, I still think it might happen" [Karen].*

The self under pressure

Infertility also needs to be seen as an individual experience. Every woman will respond differently. However, its unpredictability means that for most women it is a crisis, often with clearly identifiable stages of shock, denial, guilt, anger, depression, vulnerability and loss of identity. Additionally, infertility can be seen as a treadmill in which the infertile are beset by pressures. These were identified as the pressure of how far to pursue treatment:

"There comes a point when you have to stop. Its taken so long — you can never have different tests at the same time and they seen to do things for the sake of it. I still don't know why I had a laparoscopy. I just feel I've got to move on and I can't when I am going to the hospital every couple months" [Karen].

For many women, public explanations were the most difficult aspect of their infertility. There was the pressure exerted by family and friends:

"I feel bad for my parents, that they're getting old and aren't grandparents and all their friends are. I do feel I've failed them somehow" [Kate].

Most of the women described their response to their fertility problems as losing control not only over their body, which is not performing a basic function, but also over their life plans and ability to make changes:

"You see other people moving on and you're stuck in this kind of limbo. You hope something will happen and there will be this major change in your life, but nothing does. You might do things, get a job or something. It's just this feeling of powerlessness. You're not able to control your life" [Liz].

There is the pressure on a relationship from having 'dutiful sex' when temperature charts suggest it is a fertile period, the pressure of time passing and the pressure on one's self image:

"Women are supposed to be able to do this kind of thing. You question everything, one's own femininity as well. Like I think if I had been more womanly — if I had wanted children at twenty-two rather than thirty-five... it's taken me a long time to grow up" [Mary].

Motherhood denied

The desire for children, acknowledged as socialised by many women, was nevertheless an unquestioned and powerful drive:

"I always knew I wanted children ...it's a very basic thing... It's about having a child definitely, not just being a parent" [Karen].

"You know it isn't all there is to life but you want that as a background, as part of it" [Jean]

For several women, being childless denied them a role in society:

"Unless I have a child I won't have the same consciousness that women have who have children. I feel there will be quite a gulf between me and women who have got children" [Mary].

Women with children seem very evident to those who are childless yet, as Mary remarked:

"Whilst there are people with children and people without children, you never see people who are trying to have children" [Mary].

Infertility is rarely spoken about. One woman referred to 'hushed tones' when the subject was discussed in her family and another blamed such stigma for her own isolation:

"I knew it wasn't going to be easy but I still didn't expect it because no one ever spoke about it. Even when I'd say at work we were trying but it was taking a while and all the euphemisms you use ... people would say 'Oh, I never had any problem, a bit like falling off a log' or 'I could have done with a bit of that' " [Kate].

Health education

For the women in this study, health education should start with providing more information. Karen felt that the emphasis on unwanted pregnancies obscures the large number of couples who have difficulty conceiving:

> *"I think there should be more information aimed at the mid-twenties. If it was done sensitively enough it would be offering more choice. When you're in your twenties and doctors go on about elderly prima gravidas you just think 'stupid doctors what an appalling way to describe people' but there's nothing about the medical reasons which might lead doctors to think like that" [Karen].*

Because women do not expect to find themselves infertile, they may lack even basic information about their bodies. Karen, in common with most of the women interviewed, was unclear about ovulation and when she would be most fertile:

> *"I never knew you count back from the period you're expecting. Like I thought it was round the middle of the month but I never knew it was related to that and not fourteen days after your last period" [Karen].*

Most of the women felt the need for counselling and that this should be on an individual basis as many did not wish to be labelled as infertile or seen as part of a group:

> *"There's this assumption that we are all the same. But people are all at different stages and want different things. I think the distress people feel is so great they can't actually help each other. It's a sort of silent distress" [Jean].*

Implications for health education

The World Health Organisation estimates that between 5–10 per cent of couples in western countries may be sub fertile or infertile.

Such statistics, though widely quoted, do not provide a complete picture of infertility since they are based on women past childbearing age who do not have children. They do not take into account, therefore, the sub fertile who may eventually conceive, single women who wish to have children and those who divorce or find new partners because of one partner's infertility. Although other studies reach similar conclusions about the incidence of infertility (Hull, 1985; Johnson, 1987), the subject is rarely discussed in public perhaps because it entails the management of sexual relations or because people do not feel comfortable sharing another's grief. Infertility is not a high profile area in medicine either. Those who are conducting treatment or research are usually specialists in another area such as gynaecology or urology. The ambivalence of feminism towards motherhood which is seen by some as part of patriarchal oppression and by others as the fulfilment of being a woman has meant that infertility has been largely ignored in the women's health movement (Doyal, 1987).

As infertility is neither life threatening nor an illness but seen as a lack of a social relationship, it has a low priority in the NHS. For most people, infertility is a temporary existence which will affect large numbers for a short period of time only. The World Health Organisation estimates, for example, that 20–35 per cent of those diagnosed as having `unexplained infertility' will eventually conceive (WHO, 1985). The absence of epidemiological data makes it hard to prioritise on the basis of need and the present organisation of services is haphazard, more the result of individual consultant's interest than any Department of Health or district health authority policy. Increasingly, as Pfeffer and Quick (1988) point out in their survey of London provision, infertility treatments such as in vitro fertilisation and donor insemination have to be paid for within NHS clinics. Of the women in this study, all were undergoing investigations at London NHS hospitals having waited an average of eight months for a first appointment. Two of the women were paying for IVF treatment because the waiting list of between two and four years would put them beyond the age limit of forty imposed by most IVF units.

The hazards of reproductive technology in its physical risks, emotional upheavals and the lack of control for women have been extensively outlined elsewhere (Arditti, 1984; Corea, 1985; Lasker and Borg, 1987; Klein, 1989; Spallone, 1989). It receives disproportionate publicity to its success rates and the number of women who are able to receive such treatment, but it is not surprising that women see new technologies as 'magic solutions'. Their choice of treatment needs to be an informed one through the provision of full information, including for example, 'take-home baby rates' in the case of IVF and greater control of such technology through licensing and monitoring agencies. Change is also needed not just in the availability of services but in how those services are provided, offering more community based care which allows women the opportunity to reflect on what choices are available before they become involved in possibly lengthy and extensive investigations. One London health authority has suggested as part of their Health For All 2000 targets, that first level investigations should be carried out by GPs and counselling should be available in family planning clinics. Pfeffer and Quick (1988) suggest that key workers should be part of multi disciplinary teams based in specialist centres.

It is important that we do not ignore structural considerations in terms of causation and how women may be affected unequally by infertility. Little is known about the causes of infertility. At least 30 per cent of those who present for treatment are diagnosed as having 'unexplained infertility'. In some cases, however, infertility is known to be linked to certain preventable factors. In one study, 50 per cent of women with a history of pelvic inflammatory disease had an infection-related diagnosis and about 40 per cent of these infections are due to chlamydia bacteria. It has been estimated that using an intrauterine device doubles the risk of becoming infertile because of an infection (World Health Organisation, 1985). There is also a highly significant trend of fertility decreasing as the number of cigarettes smoked each day increases (Howe, 1985). Elkington (1986) also argues that environmental and workplace pollution presents significant reproductive hazards and are responsible for marked decreases in male sperm counts.

The notion that infertility is an individual responsibility is reinforced by available literature. Most books about pregnancy do not mention infertility or have a couple of pages on 'when you have difficulty'. One popular guide for infertile couples suggests that it is possible to help oneself conceive as 'very few couples it seems, ask themselves if there's anything that they might be doing which makes conception less likely' (Stanway, 1984). Most of the women in this study had tried to change their behaviour and frequently blamed themselves for what was perceived as a failure to conceive. However, the stress that arises from trying to change one aspect of health-damaging behaviour only exacerbated their feelings of powerlessness.

"I gave up drinking for three months but I've stopped now. It just made it worse. I was doing all that and still nothing happened" [Margaret].

Self-help recommendations, such as abstaining from intercourse before the fertile period in order to 'store up sperm', placing a pillow under the hips during intercourse to bathe the cervix in a pool of semen or adopting the missionary position for intercourse so that no sperm spill out were widely practised, although there is little basis for their effectiveness. It is important that infertility is not an opportunity for victim blaming and that such aspects of lifestyle are seen in the context of a wider society which encourages health damaging behaviour. The demand should not be for more medicine, whether preventive or curative, or new technologies but to promote the use of condoms, screening for sexually transmitted disease, the identification of reproductive hazards and programmes to help women give up smoking.

Much could also be done by health educators when working with young people to increase fertility awareness. At present, one of the main messages in young people's sex education is to prevent unwanted pregnancy and, therefore, for contraception to be taken seriously, the possibility of pregnancy being emphasised with a supposedly inevitable path of sperm to egg.

Houghton and Houghton (1984) describe infertility as 'unfocused grief'. The infertile suffer the loss of a child they can never have without the rituals of grieving. Solomon (1989) likens the experience to a crisis. All people in crisis can become dependent on whatever help is offered particularly if, as medicine, it seems to offer a solution. Each woman thus needs individual support and counselling. Working towards self-empowerment in health education means encouraging women to become more knowledgeable, to make life changes or perhaps to stop or change treatment. Pregnancy may remain the only possible solution for some women but for others, coping is a positive reaction and an alternative to treatment.

Health educators working with infertile women need to help those women identify the cultural pressures towards motherhood and see themselves other than in relation to their reproductive capacity. The public sector is uniquely placed to remove one of the barriers for infertile women, namely to make maternity rights transferable so that those experiencing fertility problems do not become attached to their place of work for seemingly indefinite periods of time for fear of losing their maternity provision. Infertility needs to be placed on the agenda of women's health education alongside the current emphasis on maternal health and women as health educators of young children in areas such as nutrition and development. Social trends indicate that 17 per cent of women born in 1955 will remain childless. Yet if women see themselves only through their relationships with children as mothers or daughters — and only such relationships can give their lives purpose, then because mothering is not open to all women, the infertile (and the voluntarily childless) are not only stigmatised but also become marginal in society.

Implications of this research

There are a number of methodological issues that arose from this research which might interest other researchers whose inquiry also seeks to be co-operative and non-hierarchical.

One of the ethical issues that confronts many researchers is the value of the research to its participants. This kind of study in which the researcher invests their personal identity, is very challenging. It means incorporating one's own experience into work and yet the researcher has to hold onto the fact that the encounter is not a conversation. It is a specialised interaction for a specific purpose. Researchers would benefit from counselling or therapeutic skills which would equip them with a balance of active listening and authenticity.

In such an intense, but nevertheless professional, encounter is there a place for involvement or friendship? Traditional forms of inquiry, work or therapeutic relationships all necessitate closure as essential for the researcher to continue their work. Three of the women, whom I had not met previously, continued in social contact as friends but also sought my support through their medical investigations. Because the numbers involved in this study were small, I was prepared for this longer term commitment. In larger studies however, it would be necessary to establish at the outset the levels of time and commitment that could be offered.

The participants in the study did find it of value although their comments do not vary significantly from those offered by participants in other forms of qualitative research that has not been set up as a shared encounter. Typical comments included:

"It made me think about it more" [Kate]

"It was really helpful to talk about it as I wanted to. It's always been pressured in other places — at the hospital or to my family" [Karen]

"It has helped me to make up my mind to stop the treatment for a while" [Margaret]

"I liked you offering things — I could define myself in relation to that, like it could be the same or different" [Mary]

For the subjects, a shared encounter is demanding. Their expectations were shaped by traditional forms of enquiry and many found it difficult to explore at length in an unfocused interview.

"I think I looked to you to give more direction. It meant I had to think about it all more and there didn't seem to be any boundaries. I didn't know if I was giving you what you wanted to know" [Karen]

It is clear to me now that I had not involved the subjects in a co-operative enquiry merely given them control over their own data. The concept of a shared encounter needed far more discussion at the outset.

For those who continue research in the area of infertility, the complexity of the experience should not be overlooked and the medical and social needs of infertile people should be addressed. Most research on infertility seeks to uncover causes or the relative success of different treatments. It draws on established frameworks of scientific inquiry and is conducted from medical establishments and it will never really take account of women's own experience and its ideological expression. The medical paradigm of infertility which focuses on biological destiny, psychological constructions of motherhood and a mechanistic view of the body has enormous influence on the meaning of infertility to women themselves. Yet infertility vividly demonstrates that health is holistic, affecting and influenced by, many aspects of the whole self including the physical.

Qualitative and descriptive approaches in health research add to scientific inquiry, offering another way of understanding.

by Jane Wills

Unfortunately, it is often seen only as a first line of investigation to produce material and ideas which will establish the basic terms of reference for a further study. It may be dismissed as `anecdotal' or `not generalisable'. Yet it can bring into medical science and the health service a more responsive, more individual viewpoint. This is especially important when `like all stigmatising conditions, infertility is made the dominant characteristic of the whole person, and fundamental differences between infertile people are ignored' (Pfeffer and Quick, 1988).

Although this study focused on women's experience, infertility is not a `woman's problem'. The focus on women and infertility as a branch of gynaecology, has had an adverse effect on treatment services which often ignore the male partner and then subject women to sometimes unnecessary and invasive tests.

If more qualitative research was available on infertility which gave a stronger voice to men and women's experience, there might emerge a more vociferous lobby around the right to have children as there has been around the choices in childbirth. Until that research is available, infertility services will continue to be badly organised and not fully integrated into the health service. They will continue to pathologise infertility, encouraging women to be victims.

References

Arditti R et al (1984) Test Tube Women: What Future for Motherhood? Pandora, London

Berer M (1985) Infertility — A Suitable Case for Treatment. Marxism Today

Chalmers AF (1982) What is this thing called science? Open University, Milton Keynes

Corea G (1985) The Mother Machine: Reproductive Technology from Artificial Insemination to Artificial Wombs. Harper Row, New York

Diczafalusy E (1986) World Health Organisation Special Programme of Research, Development and Research Training in Human Reproduction `The First Fifteen Years: A Review'. *Contraception* **34**: 1

Doyal L (1987) Unhealthy Lives: Being a Woman in London. Women's Study Unit, Polytechnic of North London

Finch J (1984) It's great to have someone to talk to: the ethics and politics of interviewing women. In: Bell C and Roberts H (eds.) *Social Researching: Politics, Problems and Practice*. Routledge and Kegan Paul, London

Glaser BG and Strauss AL (1968) *The Discovery of Grounded Theory*. Weidenfeld and Nicholson, London

Hochschild A (1975) The Sociology of Feeling and Emotion: selected possibilities. In: Millman M and Kanter (eds.) *Another Voice: Feminist Perspectives on Social Life and Social Science*. Doubleday, New York

Houghton D, Houghton P (1987) *Coping with Childlessness*. Allen Unwin, London

Howe G *et al* (1985) Effects of Age, Cigarette Smoking and other factors on fertility: findings in a large prospective study. *Br Med J* 290

Hull MGR *et al* (1985) Population study of causes, treatment and outcome of infertility. *Br Med J* 291: 1693–97

Keller EF (1983) *Gender and Science.*

Klein RD (ed) (1989) *Infertility: Women Speak Out About Their Experiences of Reproductive Medicine*. Pandora, London

Johnson G *et al* (1987) Infertile or childless by choice? A multipractice study of women aged 35 and 50. *Br Med J* 294

Mannheim K (1936) *Ideology and Utopia*. Routledge and Kegan Paul, London

Massarik F (1981) The Interviewing Process Re-examined. In: Rowan J and Reason P (eds.). Human Inquiry: *A sourcebook of New Paradigm Research*. Wiley, Chichester

Oakley A (1981) *From Here to Maternity: Becoming a Mother*. Penguin, London

Parson T (1951) *The Social System*. Free Press, New York

Pfeffer N, Woolett A (1983) *The Experience of Infertility*. Virago, London

Pfeffer N, Quick A (1988) *Infertility Services: A Desperate Case*. Greater London Association of Community Health Councils

Reason P, Hawkins (1988) Storytelling as Inquiry. In: Reason P, *Human Inquiry in Action*. Sage, London

Rowan J, Reason P (eds.) (1981) *Human Inquiry: A Sourcebook of New Paradigm Research*. Wiley, Chichester

Solomon A (1989) Infertility as crisis: Coping, Surviving — and Thriving. In: Klein RD (ed) *Op Cit*

Spallone P (1989) *Beyond Conception: The New Politics of Reproduction*. Macmillan, Basingstoke

Stainton Rogers W (1991) *Explaining Health and Illness: an exploration of diversity*. Harvester, Hemel Hempstead

Stanway A (1984) *Infertility: A Common-sense Guide for the Infertile*. Thorsons, Wellingborough

Warnock M (1985) *A Question of Life*. Blackwell, Oxford

Wills J (1989) *Women's Experience of Infertility: some shared encounters*. Unpublished dissertation, Kings College, London

Wills J (1992) Infertility: an issue for health education. *J Adv Health Nurs Care* 2: 2

World Health Organisation (1985) *Special Programme of Research Development and Research Training in Human Reproduction*. WHO, Geneva

CHAPTER FOUR
RACE, GENDER and CULTURE in SOUTH ASIAN WOMEN'S HEALTH: A STUDY in GLASGOW

A M Bowes and T M Domokos

Introduction

Studies of black women in Britain have tended to emphasise culture, 'race' or gender as factors determining their lifestyle and life chances. We will argue in this chapter that a focus on one of these factors obscures rather than illuminates understanding of black women's situation, and therefore lessens likelihood of its improvement. Our purpose is to examine the interrelationship of culture, 'race' and gender throughout the process of researching women's health, from setting out research aims through to the presentation and interpretation of research findings.

We report and discuss the process of a research project on South Asian women's health carried out in Glasgow in 1991, which proceeded from the starting point of women's own views. Instead of assuming the key health issues for South Asian women as much previous research has done, the project was designed to ask women, as users of mainstream health services, about their experiences of health services, their responses to the care received, and their views about ways of improving the services to be more appropriate and accessible for South Asian women. In their responses, the women revealed many concerns shared by other categories of women in this society, and thus showed themselves subject to the gender biases in health services experienced by all women (cf. Doyal 1985, Roberts 1985). They also revealed concerns which appeared distinctive to South Asian women, but this distinctiveness was not wholly attributable to the kinds of cultural factors stressed in much other research (detailed references are given in Bowes and Domokos 1993). It reflected significantly the process of labelling and stereotyping in this society which we call racism (see also Bowes and Domokos 1992, 1993, 1995).

Culture and South Asian health

The health care needs of South Asian women in Britain are often assumed to be distinctive, due, it is argued, to cultural differences between South Asians and the white population. Assumptions of cultural differences have seemingly dictated the subject matter of much research, so, for example, attention has been focused historically on the incidence of tuberculosis (e.g. Frogatt 1985) and rickets (e.g. Goel 1981) as particularly South Asian maladies. Several studies (e.g. Aslam *et al* 1981) have looked at traditional medicine and healers, examining the extent of their use and their potentialities for harm. Cultural practices such as the use of surma (cf Pearson 1986), diet (cf Douglas 1992) and purdah (cf Currah 1986) have been scrutinised for their dangers. Recently, this stress on culture has been criticised, both within the health research field (e.g. Rathwell and Phillips 1983, Cox and Bostock 1989, Howlett *et al* 1992) and elsewhere (Parmar 1982, Bryan *et al* 1985). Critics argue that such work assumes that South Asian culture is bad for people's health and that culture determines health status, with the result that South Asian people are being marginalised and blamed for their own health problems. Similar concerns and problems have carried over into health care initiatives and have, in many commentator's views, therefore restricted their no-doubt well-intentioned effects: two examples are the Asian Mother and Baby Campaign (Rocheron 1988 gives detailed criticism) and health education campaigns on rickets and surma (criticised in detail by Pearson 1986). Phoenix (1988) argues strongly that culture as an explanatory factor in health behaviour (in her work, teenage pregnancy) is considered relevant for black women, but not white women, thus raising the 'race' issue (see below).

An important problem in the culturally deterministic arguments is the stereotypical notion of culture they generally use. Douglas (1992) is sharply critical of this, noting that stereotyping implies homogeneity. Brah (1992: 69) refers to stereotypes of South Asian cultures thus:

> *They operate within a totally reified concept of culture as some kind of baggage to be carried around, instead of a dynamic and potentially oppositional force...*

With Lawrence (1982), she argues that South Asian cultures have been treated by `white sociology' as traditional, hidebound and backward looking.

It is necessary, we will argue, to question not only the primacy of culture as a determining and explanatory factor, but also the meaning of the concept itself. The concept needs to be stripped of stereotyping assumptions and defined, in the anthropological sense, as world view, certainly a dynamic force in Brah's (1992) terms.

Gender and 'race' in women's health research

Feminist sociologists have now been discussing issues of gender in research for several years. Writers such as Oakley (1981) and Finch (1984) particularly support the use of qualitative research methods when working with women, and their work suggests that a woman researcher can develop a special rapport with her women 'subjects' because of shared, gender-based experiences. More recently in the health field, Ramazanoglu (1990) has argued more fully that empowerment of the researched is essential to fully developed feminist sociology, and for this to be complemented by non-hierarchical, collective ways of working within research teams.

She also raises the need for disclosure by interviewers to make interviews an exchange process, rather than a one-way extraction of information, and Roberts (1992) argues for a reflexive way of working, allowing the researched to define issues as well as the researchers. Scott (1992:60) takes issue with the empowerment argument, by criticising research which disempowers and deskills the researcher, resulting in 'a lowest common denominator approach which leads to the researcher silencing herself in order to give the other project workers a voice'. Opie (1992) argues that some feminist researchers are guilty of ideological imposition in their zeal to empower the researched, because of preconceived notions of appropriate empowerment. Both Scott (1992) and Opie (1992) argue that the hallmark of feminist research is not empowerment *per se*, but the presentation of 'fissured' accounts (Opie 1992:58), in which 'the different and often competing voices within a society are recognised'.

In this feminist sociology, very little attention has been paid to issues of 'race' in the research process, and to the relationship between gender issues and 'race' issues. while Donovan (1984) describes her ethnic origin and her opposition to racism based particularly on experiences of anti-semitism, she does not reflect at length on inequalities in the interviewing process, or on the issue of different or competing voices. Douglas (1992:39) argues strongly that white women's accounts of black women's experiences are flawed because of 'the assumption that the shared experiences uniting women outweigh the differences in relation to 'race' and class'. In her view (pp40-41), 'for black women, racism is paramount': white women do not experience racism, and cannot therefore understand black women's experiences. Kazi's (1986) argument questions both Donovan's and Douglas' positions, and urges white women to drop their assumptions about what black women's problems are. She encourages black and white women to research in partnership, and to explore much more fully the complicated relationships between 'race', gender and class. Ramazanoglu (1989a, 1990) is in sympathy with this. In her work

(1989b) reappraising research on women factory workers carried out in the 1960s, she castigates herself for ignoring issues of 'race': Caribbean women workers were excluded from the study on the grounds that they would render the results statistically unreliable. The Caribbean women were not told of this. A feminist perspective, to be truly effective, would be far more conscious of 'race' issues, and would also adopt methods empowering the researched, that is allowing their voices and views to be heard. Analytically, argues Ramazanoglu (1989), there is far more work to be done on the relationships between the socially constructed phenomena of 'race' and gender and the ways they affect black and white women's lives.

Feminist research with black women as the researched therefore remains undeveloped. There is clearly a need for empirical work which will enable the strands of 'race' and gender to be unravelled, issues of empowerment in research to be explored, and 'fissured' accounts to be presented. To avoid the assumptions about culture we have criticised, to avoid the possibility of Opie's (1992) feminism imposed, and Kazi's (1986) patronising racism, it is clear that the 'fissured' account must begin with women's own views. In the account which follows, we will demonstrate that these very often challenge received 'wisdom'.

Before we begin to examine the women's statements, it is necessary to examine the study itself, and the circumstances in which, the women's views were raised. Thus we will not be presenting disembodied 'findings', but the results of a reflexive research process.

The study

Twenty South Asian Muslim women (average age 35 years) were interviewed in Glasgow in Summer 1991. Fifteen had been born in Pakistan, three in UK, one in Kenya and one in Libya. On average, they had four children, mostly of school or pre-school age. Four were single parents. Three had full-time jobs outside the home, and four, part-time jobs. In appearance, the women were traditional: all but one habitually wore the *shalwar chameez* ('Punjabi dress'), and all but four wore their hair traditionally uncut. Nearly all lived in tenemental housing in a central area of the city. The interviewees were contacted using a network of personal relationships, as local experience had shown (e.g. Bowes 1987, Wardhaugh 1990) that this was the best way of winning women's confidence and maintaining rapport in discussing often very personal matters. By referring to earlier research (Bowes *et al* 1990b), we attempted to ensure that the women were generally typical of South Asian women in Glasgow in terms of age, socioeconomic group, housing and life-cycle stage. while the three women in full-time work were rather unusual, their wide experience of professional work with South Asian women in the city was felt to be especially valuable to the study (Bowes *et al* 1990b give details of the South Asian population in Glasgow). The women we interviewed represented only one of the several South Asian heritages in Britain today. However, we describe them as 'South Asian' throughout this discussion because we feel that the general conclusions drawn would apply whatever the interviewees' particular background.

The interviews were conducted in English: in five cases, at the woman's own request, an interpreter, known to her, accompanied the interviewer. A schedule, listing topics we hoped to cover, guided the interviews, but the aim throughout was to encourage women to raise issues which they thought were particularly important, in other words, to listen to the women rather than imposing views on them (see above). Thus, all the interviews dealt with most of the topics, but each one emphasised the woman's own concerns. Interview transcripts were then coded and sorted, and produced a systematic data file organised according to the topics on the schedule and the topics the women had emphasised themselves. The main areas of discussion were health and health maintenance, the life cycle, illness, children, the use of health services and alternatives, non-professional help and support given and received, and the environment. Some topics proved more sensitive, particularly breast feeding, breast cancer and childbirth, whereas others, notably cervical smear tests and personal relationships, were less problematic than we had anticipated (More detail on the approach appears in Bowes and Domokos 1992).

The researchers

We (Bowes and Domokos) are both female, mature, mothers, older than the average woman interviewed. Domokos, who did most of the fieldwork, is an experienced nurse, midwife and counsellor. Bowes has formal research training and experience, including work with women in kibbutzim (Bowes 1978, 1986) and with South Asians in Glasgow (Bowes 1987, Bowes, McCluskey and Sim 1990a, 1990b, 1990c). Our social positions should have been assets, allowing Oakley's (1981) shared experiences and Finch's (1984) easy rapport, and indeed we found most of the women to be very open, to welcome the chance to talk. They gave us large pieces of their time and space, as most of the interviews were in their homes. Our professional research training and experience were also important assets: we would not denigrate academic skills, or silence them to find the 'lowest common denominator' (Scott 1992). Domokos' nursing background proved crucial in realising what had happened to some of the women interviewed in encounters with health services: she was able to see how in several cases, hospital procedures had been followed without regard for women's communication difficulties, and women had been left mystified by the whole experience. For example, one woman in particular was frightened to return to a consultant regarding her asthma treatment because using the peak flow meter (a test, described by the woman concerned as an unnamed 'treatment') made her breathless. She complained that the doctor did not listen when she tried to say the 'treatment' upset her.

As well as looking at the women's statements in analysing the interviews, we also looked at the interviewer's comments. We used a non-directive form of interviewing, designed to allow women to express their own views, and the role of the interviewer was to encourage women to comment on the areas covered by the checklist, and to support them in doing so. Ramazanoglu (1990) comments extensively on the counselling which became involved in some of the Women Risk and Aids Project (WRAP) team's interviews with young women about their sexuality, which became particularly significant where young women revealed, sometimes for the first time, experiences of sexual abuse. In our interviews, we also encountered situations where counselling became relevant, such as talk of recent, painful bereavement and relationship problems. In one case, Domokos was asked to return for a further talk, and agreed to do so.

Monitoring Domokos' supporting comments (apart from questions) during interviews, these fall roughly into three categories. Some are simply support to the woman, such as

You must be very busy, going to the hospital so often

or

It's difficult to rest when you're changing house isn't it?

or

It must have been difficult when the children were small

Support was also communicated in non-verbal ways, including, the physical set up of the interviews, and the interviewer's attention to the woman. The transcripts show frequent use of `Mmmm' in several supporting and encouraging variations.

A second category of comments involves self-disclosure (an issue also raised by Ramazanoglu (1990)):

'I'm from a large family ... but I've only got two children myself.
I'm not as strong as my mother was'

Bowes also did this

'My father has an ulcer as well, and he was told to eat little and often. He says it's better — he eats all the time.'

The third category of comment was responses to requests for advice.

'It's good to sit down and do some deep breathing and try to relax before you feed the child.'

'She doesn't need to wait until she has sex to improve it [daughter's period pain]: she can have some treatment for it.'

'No, for the diabetes there isn't a cure, it just has to be managed, stabilised.'

We considered it a responsibility, having invaded our interviewees' lives, to be able to respond to their requests to us, by being prepared to accept counselling as part of the interviewing process, by giving straightforward medical information, and by giving information about sources of advice and treatment (cf Ramazanoglu 1990).

All the points discussed here were important to the good rapport which allowed the interviews to go well, that is, for the objective of ascertaining women's own points of view, to be achieved. But there is a further important factor which must be examined, the factor of 'race'. Both researchers are white, and therefore could not share experiences of racism with the women interviewed. We can both recount experiences of ethnic prejudice (which Anthias and Yuval-Davis 1983 have argued parallels racism), but must concur with Kazi (1986) that racism experienced by South Asian women in Britain is qualitatively different. This is because of the social structural correlates of racism, particularly those linked to power, which mean that white people benefit from it, for example by having black people do many of the most menial jobs in society because of a distinct employment structure.

If we were to accept (as Douglas 1992 apparently argues) that research is impossible without shared experience, then most research would be rendered pointless. To take the other extreme and argue that experiences make no difference, would in this context deny the very trenchant criticisms of 'white sociology' (Lawrence 1982) and its neglect of issues of gender and 'race', and also the criticisms of feminist sociology (above) concerning its assumptions about the supremacy of gender and its general ignorance of issues of 'race' and racism. As we see it, the point is to be open to the experiences of the researched, not to predefine them, or interpret them according to any ideological preconceptions. In particular, researchers must listen for challenges to their own expectations and assumptions. For white women working with black women, 'race' is a key area in which these challenges may be found. It is not the only area, as we will show.

In conducting the research, we were aware of the problems of stereotyping minority cultures (noted above). It was important to be sensitive to the women's culture, in the anthropological sense of world view, without assuming what it was. We noted (above) with reference to Phoenix (1988) that culture is often seen as an issue in research about black women, but not generally in research about white women, reflecting the society wide construction of black women as 'other' (cf Miles 1989), which is part of racism.

The interviews were transcribed, and then coded, to allow us to find our way around the several hundred pages of typescript generated. The coding system we used was very simple, and used the topics from the interview schedule initially. Topics which the women had raised were also given codes as they emerged from the transcripts. We restricted the coding to fifty topics, allowing these to be divided into subtopics if this made the material easier to handle. For example the topic `childbirth' was divided into `family size' `preparation for childbirth' `maternity care' `breast feeding' `places of birth' and `general' (for comments that did not fit elsewhere). The codes were attached to whole paragraphs, to preserve some contextual comments, and included references to the original transcripts to make it easy to look back to these. Paragraphs could be given more than one code, if they covered several topics. To allocate the codes, the transcripts were read and annotated with topics, and the codes themselves added after a second reading. To ensure reasonable consistency, we did some independently, then compared notes afterwards: we found our coding was consistent, probably because the scheme itself was simple.

The sorting procedure produced files which contained, for example, everything that had been said about preparation for childbirth, labelled by interview. Such a file allowed the range of comments to be easily seen, any quantifiable data to be extracted, and reference back to the original transcripts to be made.

We deliberately adopted this straightforward scheme for organising data because of our desire to reflect the women's own views. The scheme allowed constant reference back to the transcripts during writing, and this meant that we maintained sight of the context in which comments had been made, including the circumstances of the interview and the characteristics of the woman speaking (which were noted separately). Thus the findings were less likely to become disembodied, processed data, possibly out of touch with reality due to being overworked through complex classification. The self-imposed restriction on the number of categories we used was also intended to help prevent over-elaboration. We see one of the main advantages of this method of analysing data to be the constant reminders it generates of the inconsistencies and competing voices which must become part of the fissured account. Some of these voices are those of the researchers: it is also important that we were made repeatedly aware of the coding we had done, through the constant references back to the original transcripts, and that the coding did not therefore become reified.

Key issues in South Asian women's health

In the interviews, women's own views of what were important health matters differed very markedly from the concerns of the stereotyping, culturally deterministic research we criticised. In this section of the paper we take three issues discussed in the interviews, and discuss them in the context of current health service provision, examining the interplay of factors of culture, gender and 'race'. The three issues are selected firstly, on the grounds that they were widely discussed by the women and were therefore important for them, and secondly, because they allow us to examine culture, gender and `race', with reference to the way others have used these factors to generate explanations. The issues are firstly, cervical cytology in which the role of cultural factors is often stressed; secondly, childbirth, which feminists have constructed primarily as a gender issue; and thirdly, racism, which has been seen by some as the primary determinant of South Asian women's lives in Britain. In some respects, South Asian women's views about and experiences related to these areas are similar to those of other women: here the shared gender dimensions are important. In other respects, their views and experiences are different: sometimes, cultural factors come into play here, but there are also strong indications that the 'race' factor, constructed as racism, is a crucial process shaping women's views and experiences.

Cervical cytology — a cultural taboo?

We specifically asked women about health checks in the interviews, framing questions in a general way, partly because of the general intention to allow women's own views to emerge, but also because, although this was an important area of interest for us, we suspected that women might be embarrassed by direct questioning about the cervical smear test. Nine women were keen for general health checks to be available, and six volunteered that they had recently had the smear test. Two of the professional workers reported that the special testing sessions they had arranged locally for South Asian women had proved very popular: their efforts had responded to local concern that women were not having their tests. We found no embarrassment attached to the subject discussed in this way (with, importantly we think, a mature married woman), and the women were generally very positive about this aspect of preventive medicine:

I think it's good that they're looking after you. That they care for you, you know like say, if there's anything wrong, they could find it quick and treat it.

There were also indications that some women did not want to be tested, because they did not want to know of any problems: this attitude has also been noted among non-Asian women (e.g. McKie *et al* 1990). One woman we interviewed had been recalled after a smear:

She asked me to come up again, and I [didn't go] again.

This woman went on to explain that she had been frightened by the request for a repeat smear, and that if there was anything wrong, she would prefer not to know.

In terms of objective risk, there is some disturbing, though tentative, evidence that the rate of cervical cancer among South Asian women in the West of Scotland may be four times that for other women (Matheson *et al* 1985). while women we interviewed certainly saw the cervical smear test as important (here they differed from many South Asian women — McAvoy and Raza 1988), there was no indication that they were aware of a greater than average risk of cancer.

In the West of Scotland, breast cancer is a far more significant killer of women than cervical cancer (Greater Glasgow Health Board 1990). The incidence of the disease has been found to be lower among women in the Indian subcontinent, though of earlier onset (McAvoy 1990). It is unknown whether the rate for South Asian women in Britain is now reaching that for non-Asians, as has happened historically in other populations of immigrant origin (McAvoy 1990). Despite the greater objective problems for women posed by breast cancer, the topic was raised by only one of the women interviewed in connection with health checks. She spoke about the local screening programme, suggesting that women would be keen to participate:

Breast screening — that's what people are asking for.

Cervical and breast cancer are certainly key health issues for all women, including South Asian women. In that respect, shared gender is undoubtedly important. There is some evidence that South Asian women's objective risks are distinctive, but no clear indications that their attitudes to tests are consistent and culturally dictated. For example, a culturally focused interpretation of our material might argue that women did not discuss breast cancer, screening, breast awareness or self-examination (all topics of recent widespread media discussion), because of some culturally dictated taboo on the breast. Some of the comments on breast feeding might be used to support this, as well as the rather low rates of breast feeding. In our view, such an interpretation would be seriously misleading. If South Asian women are compared with women in the general Glasgow population, the rate of breast-feeding (defined as any attempt to do so) is much higher, at 50 per cent overall (GGHB 1989), compared with 30 per cent for white women (GGHB 1989), a rate reducing to about 18 per cent for the most deprived areas (GGHB 1990). The Greater Glasgow Health Board's breast screening programme, which commenced in 1988, aimed to cover all women aged 50-64 in the Board area by 1993 (GGHB 1989). Thus not only were the women interviewed living in a largely non-breast feeding environment, but also, as far as the local breast cancer detection campaign was concerned, they were excluded on the grounds of age. There is no reason to assume these environmental factors to be irrelevant for South Asian women, and there is certainly scope for much more detailed research in this area.

Such an argument for the significance of environmental facts is further supported by consideration of the issues relating to cervical cytology. Whereas other research (e.g. McKie *et al* 1990) has been nervous about approaching South Asian women about this topic, and we were also worried about embarrassing women, our fears, as we have noted, proved unfounded. while it is important to take account of the sensibilities of those researched, there is a danger that women may be excluded from important areas of research, and their voices remain unheard because of an over-cautious approach. Such excessive caution is far more likely, we would argue, for categories of women, such as South Asian women, who are socially constructed as distinct, by virtue of their culture, or their position in society. Hence, environmental factors can dictate research issues in this way, and feminist researchers can become paralysed by their attempts to be sensitive to women's diverse experiences and views of the world.

Assumptions of cultural distinctiveness are, we have argued, problematic, and so is failure to ask questions on certain topics. Another important point which we argued earlier, is that researchers must listen to all the voices of the researched, if they aim to discover the full range of their views. The fissured account reveals variation rather than cultural consistency. The women interviewed were, as we have said, positive about the smear test, with some exceptions. We also noted that two of the professional workers had organised special testing sessions for local South Asian women. Again, we might argue that the impetus for this was cultural, that a distinct group of women felt different from other women, and required a special appeal, an all-female staffed session and so on. Certainly such factors were mentioned by the women who organised the sessions. But again, the information has to be put in its broader context, particularly that of women's criticisms of the difficulty of travelling to doctors' surgeries with small children on public transport, the difficulty of getting appointments, the long waits and so on. Clearly general services had their problems for the women interviewed, and the popularity of the special sessions may therefore be explained by factors relating to other service provision rather than women's particular characteristics. There seem to be generalised service failures which would affect all women, particularly those with young children, and which would influence their ability to attend for screening.

There is little evidence of attempts by the Health Board to target South Asian women, or to provide appropriate provision for them. For example, while Annual Reports (GGHB 1989,1990,1991-2) provide separate statistical information for ethnic minorities, there is no concerted consideration of possible needs for special provision for, or targeting of, South Asians, Furthermore, the recently opened women's health centre in Glasgow advertised special provision for deaf and disabled women, but the publicity offered no particular attractions for women of minority ethnic origin. While we were carrying out the research in 1991, Domokos attended one of the public meetings concerned with the establishment of the Centre: although the meeting was held in one of the main South Asian areas in the city, local South Asian groups had not been contacted directly about it, and the women we were talking to generally knew nothing about it. The one South Asian woman who attended the meeting (having been told about it by Domokos) appeared very marginal to the proceedings, partly because she was the only South Asian woman there, and partly because no translation facilities were available, and she had particular difficulties with English. All these factors suggest the Health Board has at best some way to go in its approach to South Asian women's health, and at worst is simply unaware of the need to consider the appropriateness of its own practices for this section of its clientele. It might be argued that this failure expresses institutional racism, in that the public face of the organisation does not appear to recognise that some of its practices effectively exclude South Asian women, and deny them access to certain health resources. This reflects and helps reproduce the more widespread patterns for exclusion of racialised groups in this society, known as racism (Miles 1989). In this case, we observe racism by omission, that is, an apparent failure to think through the implication of differentials between ethnic categories recorded in the Board's own statistics, and consequent failure to offer accessible services. More recently, the Board has begun to consider these issues, and (1995) is pursuing several initiatives, including the establishment of a linkworker scheme. Interwoven with this is a gender issue: as we noted, many women's problems with clinic attendance were linked to accessibility problems shared by all women with young children, and without their own transport. Thus health provision in Glasgow also lacks user-friendliness for another, overlapping category of women.

Experiences of childbirth: violence against women?

Childbirth has been and continues to be an important topic for research on women's health (Roberts 1992), and both feminist researchers (especially Oakley 1980, Kitzinger 1992) and campaigning organisations such as the National Childbirth Trust and the Association of Radical Midwives have long campaigned against the medicalisation of childbirth and for 'woman-centred and woman-controlled reproductive care' (Oakley 1980:296). Recent policy seems to be moving some way towards satisfying these demands (Health Committee Report 1991–2). Throughout research, campaigning and policy, there has been a considerable stress on gender issues.

However, other findings have suggested that black women in this society are subject to pressures additional to those on white women experiencing pregnancy and childbirth: Phoenix (1988) for example reports that health professionals often assume black women's pregnancies to be unintentional, and that they need help with birth control, suggesting effective restriction of women's choice to have babies at all, never mind how to have them. Douglas (1992:37) is critical of perspectives on Asian women which have been concerned primarily with perinatal mortality, infant mortality and low birth-weight babies, with a tendency to attribute high perinatal and infant mortality to cultural practices, lack of uptake of antenatal services and diet, rather than to maternal and economic deprivation. She sees this 'victim-blaming', focused on minority culture, as an expression of racism.

Using the non-directive interviewing technique meant that we did not press women to talk in detail about their experiences of childbirth: Kitzinger (1992) likens many women's experiences of childbirth to a form of rape, and stresses the resulting difficulty of recounting and coming to terms with them. We felt it inappropriate to press women to distress by insisting on detail in this area.

We found that women's experiences of childbirth were not in general happy memories, eagerly recalled. For many, fear was a strong element:

Yes, it is very, very frightening.

She remembered 'I'm so frightened' [translator]

Some people, they went to hospital and had awful experiences.

Three women explained they had had no preparation for pregnancy or childbirth. They had all eventually attended for antenatal care, but had not had access to antenatal classes. Several women had had caesarean sections: one in particular, who had had three, expressed bewilderment about the reasons for the operations, despite her best efforts to ask for explanations:

... they told me I had a contracted pelvis or something, too small ... I really thought it was maybe because I'm not tall in height and that, but they just said I had a pelvis too small, that's it ... it was kind of hush hush stuff, nobody actually talked about it.

Other women talked about pain. They were glad of the pain relief available.

I just didn't want to have any pain, and that was it.

In my own country, it was very, very painful, you know, they don't have gas and these kinds of things.

Some felt pain had not received proper treatment:

[The midwife] was shouting at my sister-in-law, because when, you know, when the contractions were coming, she was

screaming a little bit. Maybe it was a bit more than, you know, you'd do, but this lady pinched her, actually pinched her.

(This woman had accompanied her sister-in-law in labour)

... all night, my goodness, then morning time, he was born

(speaking of a night of pain)

Many women had negative comments about the post-natal care they had received. One spoke of her wish to stay longer in hospital:

I like to stay two or three more days at hospital because you know I'm very tired, and my husband was busy ... and she [nurse] said to me 'No, go home'. I don't know why I can't stay in hospital.

By far the most common complaint was about hospital food, particularly the lack of halal food or acceptable vegetarian alternatives. Twelve women commented unfavourably on hospital food, and many had had food brought in for them:

... the other patients, they eat, but me, just salad. Friends, they bring me food from outside, and my husband, he brought me food.

I like cheese, I like vegetables, but not all the time, you know, the same thing.

Some hospital staff expected women to receive food from outside, but this was not always practical:

She [the nurse] was saying 'why don't you phone your husband to bring something for yourself, from your family?' I said 'I've no family here'.

Other women complained about the treatment they had received from staff in other contexts:

They help the others, the Scotswomen. When I told her 'I'm very ill, could you make the bath for the baby' or something, 'Change the nappy yourself' she said to me.

The comments regarding lack of explanation, and intolerance of cries of pain (above) also reflect negative assessments of staff behaviour.

Alongside these negative accounts must be set some very positive ones, referring to all stages of the processes of pregnancy, delivery and post partum care.

With such a range of topics and relatively small number of women, it would be rash to weigh the positive and negative comments. In general, a woman's account would include comments on both sides: there were few women who gave either a wholly positive or wholly negative account. As we have commented on the particular referents of the negative comments, we can also observe patterns in the positive ones. Typical positive comments were:

I found them great, because when I was having the second child, they let me take the older child ... The doctors were great with the older one, letting her feel the baby, showing her where it is and letting her hear the heartbeat.

In the labour rooms, very good service and very, very good to babies.

... we used to be there for one week and the nurses used to look after the children at night-time as well, and you had a good night's sleep ... it was great.

... they took care of my daughter first four nights, and they didn't wake me up. I was supposed to be breast feeding her, but they helped me so much you know, so that was a big comfort.

The nurses were great, and I used to write my mum 'They're angels over here, and they don't consider if you're a black or white person'.

Throughout these comments, and indeed throughout the interviews, there was little sense of choice in childbirth in the senses stressed by the Health Committee Report (1991-2) or childbirth campaigns. Such matters as consistency of care, negotiation of pain relief, preferences for one or other birth environment were simply non-issues. Where choices were expressed, these were related to hospital conditions (especially food), the length of stay in hospital and the behaviour of staff. In the positive comments, there was a stress on staff attitudes and on levels of comfort in hospital. We suspect that choice in childbirth in the campaigning and policy sense is as much a fable for women generally as it appeared to be for the women interviewed, and that South Asian women, like others, are still generally experiencing medically managed and controlled childbirths, with care which is neither 'woman-centred' nor 'woman-controlled' (Oakley 1980:296). Furthermore, some of the negative comments made in the interviews reflect some of the violence of childbirth: the fear, the shock, the lack of explanation, the pain, all echo the comments reported by Kitzinger (1992). In these respects, women's experience was a function of society-wide gender relationships reflected in childbirth, and was clearly shared with other women in the same society.

It is also noteworthy that the positive comments related strongly to the child centred approach of the staff, and to the fact that babies were not constantly at their mothers' sides. We should add that staff overnight care of babies is widely considered detrimental to the establishment of breast feeding and to the mother-child relationship (e.g. Stanway and Stanway 1984). None of these factors qualifies as 'woman-centred' or 'woman-controlled' and all have been criticised by choice in childbirth campaigners (e.g. Stanway and Stanway 1984). The women's comments thus challenge elements of the radical childbirth movement's notions of what women want. Indeed, when elements of our analysis were presented to an anonymous referee, we were accused of being male, presumably on the grounds that only men interpreted women's comments on childbirth in a non 'woman-centred' way. In response to this criticism, we returned to the interviews and re-examined them, and concluded that our presentation had indeed reflected women's views, both negative and positive. We must re-emphasise (following Opie 1992) that our interest lies in how women actually see and experience the world, not how they ought to see and experience it.

The interviews in general and some of the comments we have reported include indications that women felt they had or had not been treated differently because of their ethnic origins or their 'race'. In commenting in this way, saying that 'Asian women' did not eat hospital food, or go to antenatal classes, or get help from hospital staff, or were treated the same as all women, the women were reflecting boundaries of great social and structural significance to the wider society around them, constructed by that society as boundaries of 'race'. Sometimes, women appeared to blame themselves for their difficulties, particularly by commenting that they could not understand what was happening to them because their English was not good enough: set against the comments of women whose English was fluent, who also complained of lack of information, this self-blame must certainly be questioned. We must conclude that although lack of information is a general problem experienced by women in childbirth, and is therefore a gender issue, for South Asian women, the apparent failure to recognise language difficulties and to provide necessary translation facilities creates an additional barrier to communication. Similarly, the non-supply of appropriate food, and the assumptions about the South Asian family structure allowing for food to be brought into hospital, indicate that South Asian women are made to face difficulties which do not confront other women. Some of the hospital practices therefore have racist effects, even though, again, this is by omission rather than commission, because they alter the access of a particular category of women to appropriate services. In some respects, South Asian women's special needs do derive from South Asian culture (such as language assistance, dietary preferences, and Rocheron *et al* 1989 mention prayer facilities and length of dressing gowns) but the non-response to these needs, and the problematic staff attitudes are functions of the hospital regime, and the culture of that regime.

Racism: the key issue?

Racism in the health service has been noted in other studies (such as Rathwell and Phillips 1983, Cox and Bostock 1989), but its specific effects and clients' experiences of it have been neglected (cf Bryan *et al* 1985). Yet, as we noted earlier, many writers argue that racism is the basis of black women's experiences in Britain. Looking at our data, and contextualising it in the wider social structure, we will argue that racism is certainly important, but would take issue with those who see it as the primary determining factor in all respects. As an emphasis on culture can obscure gender and 'race', as gender focused arguments tend to ignore 'race' and culture, so the insistence on racism as paramount prevents examination of other factors. We will suggest that an argument which can demonstrate where racism comes into play, and how it is interwoven with the other factors under discussion makes a far stronger case for tackling racism than the rather crude notion that the world is governed by racism.

The women we interviewed varied greatly in their views on racism, though it was recognised as an issue by most of them. One asked for the tape recorder to be switched off while she talked about experiences of racism. Others were very 'up-front', and urged us strongly to see racism as a primary factor.

Some women spoke of experiences more akin to Anthias and Yuval-Davis' (1983) 'ethnic prejudice' perceiving differential treatment on the basis of their cultural background. We have already presented examples of talk of this kind in the previous section, in the complaints about hospital food, and lack of translation facilities. We would argue that, although perhaps not experienced as such, these aspects in fact reflected institutional racism.

Some women spoke of racism as an everyday experience, of varying seriousness. This woman had not experienced racism as a big issue:

> *... I've never actually had any kind of extreme thing happening to me, maybe getting a name called here and there, but that's it.*

By contrast, another found herself and her children the constant victims of harassment and violence, threatened and actual:

> *I came seven o'clock night time last week ... seven or eight boys were outside of here. They throw their stone ... They don't want Asian people here.*

Two women talked of racism affecting them personally, but linked their comments into a much broader analysis, arguing that racism fundamentally shaped black women's interactions with health services, and that it affected all Asian peoples' health. One of these women looked at her own experience.

> *It affects my health ... I have to work twice as hard being black ... You have to work twice as hard, ten times as hard to be healthy as a white person.*

Then she related this to Asian people generally:

> *I'd say the present, like, racist structure affects the health of Asian people, black people. And this thing about equal opportunities in a multi-cultural society, it doesn't exist.*

The other woman focused particularly on the attitudes of health service personnel. Speaking of a job she had had, which included accompanying women on clinic visits, she recounted

> *I won't blame everybody, but some of the time it was really bad. It's just, you know, they don't see black people as human sometimes ... They're second grade citizens sometimes because they are treated like that.*

Women's responses to experiences of racism also varied. Some were philosophical about it

> *You really kind of expect things like that anyway, so you just take it in your stride.*

Talking about her job (see above) one woman said

*I used to always try to combat that in my own way. Maybe at
times I was wrong, maybe at times I was right ... I used to say
'You shouldn't be talking to people like that'.*

The other woman who saw racism as fundamental to black
women's experience explained that she wore the *shalwar chameez*
partly as a political statement, to challenge white people's
stereotypes:

*I will wear these clothes, and open my mouth later on to shock
people - you know, shock white people, because they think this is
an idiot sitting there wearing these clothes.*

Thus the interview material shows that women varied considerably
in their experiences and assessments of racism. The variation can be
related to individual biography to some extent, in that assessments
of the importance of racism relate quite closely to the degree of
direct experience of it, and to the extent to which women
contextualised these experiences with reference to wider social
processes. In these terms, only a small minority of the women
interviewed saw racism as fundamental, and, in general, those who
did so were referring to institutional rather than interpersonal
racism.

References to individual biography however enable us to
make only partial sense of these women's experiences of and
responses to racism. Their accounts have to be interpreted in the
context of the particular ideological and structural racism relating
to South Asian women in Britain today. As Brah (1992) outlines,
South Asian women are constructed as a distinctive category (called
'Paki') and are stereotyped as passive, oppressed within the South
Asian family, and sexually available, while at the same time, dirty
and undesirable, The structural dimension of what she calls
'patriarchal racism' pervades every aspect of social structure. Brah
focuses on racism in employment and education. This context
would suggest the considerable power of racism in shaping
women's experiences. But at the same time, as we have shown, and
as Brah argues, the gender dimension operates very powerfully as

well. South Asian women thus face a double burden, of sexism and racism.

White women being called for, or presenting themselves for cervical smear tests experience certain difficulties. Some of these are practical difficulties relating for example to the timing of appropriate clinics, or travel problems (cf McKie *et al* 1990). Others may be experienced as personal difficulties, such as embarrassment at being attended to by a male doctor, a sense of shame and indignity at the whole procedure, linked to their sexuality (cf McKie *et al* 1990). Others fear either the test itself, or the possibility of a positive result. Many of these problems and views can be related to the social construction of gender, and to the society-wide structural subordination of women. South Asian women, we have argued, face extra problems. Access to testing is problematic because of institutional racism, which means services are not truly ethnically sensitive. Where services and commentators do consider South Asian women perhaps to have a distinct world view, this can act to women's detriment, in that their cultural predilections are assumed to deter them from having the test.

A white woman facing childbirth for the first time is made sharply aware of the lack of control she has over the whole process. The medicalisation of childbirth compounds the general disempowerment which the woman has experienced throughout her life. The message received by the woman is that she is, after all, a baby-producing machine, to be manipulated (Kitzinger 1992) into performing her allotted function in the scheme of production and reproduction (cf Martin 1989). The South Asian woman in the same situation receives all these messages and more, which are transmitted through racism. So childbirth may be her destiny, but she will be expected to reappear too often, because South Asian women, it is believed, have too many children out of ignorance. She will likely receive the messages about being a 'second class citizen', which she will be accustomed to because 'you really kind of expect things like that anyway'. Stereotypes of South Asian family structure may ensure that little effort is made to feed her in hospital: racism is here expressed as a cultural stereotype. Genuine cultural differences may add to her disempowerment: in particular, language difficulties not catered for by the hospital will render her experience bewildering, even incomprehensible, and make her attempts to ask questions or to request help ineffective.

Thus in these situations, the dimensions of gender, 'race' and culture interweave. The particular significance of the 'race' factor is that racism is an experience faced only by women who belong to racialised groups (in this society, black women), and a structuring principle which affects only them. In these examples, it increases the effects of gender processes, working in the same direction of disempowerment. Racism uses cultural stereotypes as one of its means of operating. The effect of cultural factors truly distinctive to South Asian women is again shown to be relatively minor.

In the end, there is little point in arguing, in absolutist terms, about the relative strength of one or other factor as explaining the experiences of South Asian women. It is far more important, in our view, to demonstrate how 'race', gender and culture interweave with one another, and, as we have argued, combine to produce a strong disempowering effect.

Research has an important role to play in the challenge to racism in the health service. Examining women's experiences of racism, that is, the operation of prejudice based on purported racial identity, must have a high priority. Analytically, it is crucial to disentangle exactly where racism is operating and where other problems, such as gender bias, are being placed under the heading. A case against racism is weakened unless its operation is precisely demonstrated, and if racism is seen as a catch-all explanation for all bad experiences of health services: such an argument would be equivalent to assuming language to be the key to all communication problems, and would similarly exoticise South Asian women, assuming that their difficulties with health services arose from their distinctive attributes and not from the nature of health services. Cultural stereotyping is in itself a form of racism.

Conclusion

Our research, while on a small scale, strongly suggests that key health issues for South Asian women are not those pinpointed by cultural stereotyping or, indeed, by much previous research. Issues stressed by our interviewees were in general similar to those raised by other, particularly women, health service users. Racism was a distinct issue, but did not arise from South Asian cultures. South Asian women appear from the work most characteristically as ordinary health service consumers with ordinary problems. Their needs therefore are not radically different, but the means of satisfying them need improvement.

The fissured account demonstrates South Asian women challenging received wisdom in sociology and feminism. For sociology, they question the culturally stereotyping notions of 'health needs', and for feminism and feminist sociology, they challenge the insistence on the primacy of gender and the purported homogeneity of the category 'women'. Furthermore, and somewhat contrary to various criticisms of 'white sociology' and homogenising feminism, they also question the primacy of racism in shaping black women's lives. In each of the three areas we have examined, cervical cytology, childbirth and racism, we have argued that to make sense of women's experiences, the three aspects of culture, 'race' and gender must all be examined, and we have attempted to expose some of the complexities of their interactive influences on women's lives.

The other important contextualising dimension concerns the circumstances under which the women's accounts of their experiences were gathered, i.e. the way the research was done, which has been a particular preoccupation of writers of feminist sociology. We adopted the approach outlined with the aim of reaching, in the circumstances, women's best accounts of their experiences and views of the world, expressed in ways most satisfying to the women themselves. To achieve this aim, we tried to ensure good rapport, and to help women feel comfortable with the interviewing process. With Ramazanoglu (1989b) we would argue that any picture of the world offered by data of this kind is bound to be partial: it is important for sociological studies to reveal the factors which may be operating to obscure certain parts of the view or to bring others particularly sharply into focus. In our case, we saw our age, motherhood and professional backgrounds as advantageous, facilitating discussion of more intimate, personal areas of women's lives. With Wardhaugh (1989) we would argue that a white woman working with black women faces particular challenges, but also some advantage. The challenge is that as a white woman in a racist society, she is in a position of power vis à vis black women, additional to power deriving from her professional position, which is partly a function of class: she must be alert to the ways in which the interviewing process may reflect this power structure, and what the consequences of this may be. Furthermore, the white interviewer cannot share experiences of racism with black interviewees, and this may compound the difficulties. The advantage is that a white woman is an outsider, and many women stated that they found it easier to talk with someone who was not involved in local gossip.

In the end, every piece of data gathering must be a compromise between the perfect and the possible. What is important to the fissured account, is that the imperfections in the data gathering approach, that is, its own fissures, are revealed, as part of the general revelation of competing voices.

These conclusions have far-reaching consequences for future research on women's health at all stages in the process. They suggest a need to review the questions being asked: if we are interested in ascertaining women's own views about their health and about health services, there is little point in predetermining the nature of women's concerns, such as by assuming their preferences in childbirth, or culturally based taboos on cervical smear tests or breast examination. In the case of South Asian women (and other women racialised in this society) the dangers are twofold, in that not only are they subjected to gender stereotyping (both radical and conservative), but also they are culturally stereotyped, as we have argued. Women's world views require empirical investigation, not predetermination.

In terms of research methods, we have argued for a more reflexive way of working, firstly in the sense of being more responsive to the people being researched, and, secondly, in the sense of greater self-consciousness on the part of researchers, who need to write themselves into the presentation of research findings. while feminist researchers have made considerable progress in this area, and social anthropologists have also been debating the issues for some time (e.g. Clifford and Marcus 1986), their debates have still to spread widely through Sociological work generally.

Explanations of research findings often gloss over the richness and variability of the findings by resorting to deterministic argument. In the material we have reviewed, there has been a tendency to stress culture (viewed stereotypically) or gender or 'race' as a paramount factor accounting for aspects of South Asian women's health. We have argued that these factors interweave, and that the discovery of how they do so is a problem requiring further examination and discussion. Interpretation of research findings needs to be much more prepared to appreciate their complexity, and to avoid the reductionism entailed in single-factor explanations.

Our work has an important transformative dimension. The purpose of recounting and interpreting South Asian women's experiences of health services is to identify areas where such women are not receiving adequate service, and to demonstrate what kinds of changes will be needed to improve their rightful access to the services available for all.

Our argument against cultural stereotyping, and for the relative unimportance of cultural distinctiveness might lead to the facile conclusion that health services need to be 'colour-blind', to offer health care to all, regardless of 'race', creed or colour in an undifferentiated fashion. Such an argument would be against special provision for any category such as South Asians, or women. This type of approach, however, is characteristically detrimental to disadvantaged groups, because their disadvantage is not recognised, and institutions are absolved from self-examination of their own, albeit unwittingly, discriminatory practice. Ethnically-sensitive practice, by contrast, involves continuous awareness of the needs of particular clients, and a constant process of improvement. For example, it is important that stereotyping is recognised, and challenged, and that assumptions which arise about people's needs are constantly questioned: thus the assumption of language problems or the availability of extended family help will not mask unmet or unvoiced needs. In individual encounters, it is important to be sensitive to health service users' particular needs and wishes: for example, South Asian women may place high value on modesty, as indeed may many other women. Again, a stereotype can only prevent consideration of and sensitivity to the individual woman. A further example of ethnically sensitive practice would entail working to ensure true universal access to health services, and to reasonable choice within such access, including, for example, availability of female staff to women (and male staff to men) who want them, and availability of health promotional material on all topics, not simply those thought suitable for different client groups (cf Bhopal and Donaldson 1988, Howlett *et al* 1992), such as contraceptive advice for black women. The principles of ethnically sensitive practice, which involves an appreciation of different world views are not dissimilar from principles which would govern gender-sensitive practice.

All such strategies entail challenging racism, the one clearly distinctive aspect of the relationship between South Asian women and health services.

References

Anthias F, Yuval-Davis N (1983). 'Contextualising feminism — gender, ethnic and class divisions' *Fem Rev*, **15**: 62–75

Bowes AM (1978). 'Women in the kibbutz movement' *Sociolog Rev* **26**(2): 237–262

Bowes AM (1986) 'Israeli kibbutz women: conflict in Utopia' In: Ridd R, Callaway H (eds) *Caught up in Conflict: Women's Responses to Political Strife*. Macmillan, London: pp138-162

Bowes AM (ed) (1987) *Asian Women in Glasgow*. Crossroads Youth and Community Association, Glasgow

Bowes AM, Domokos TM (1992) *Asian Women and Health in Scotland*. Scottish Home and Health Department, Edinburgh:

Bowes AM, Domokos TM (1993) 'South Asian women and health services: a study in Glasgow' *New Community* **19** (4): 611–26

Bowes AM, Domokos TM (1995) 'Key issues in South Asian women's health: a study in Glasgow'. *Social Sci Health* **1** (3): 145–57

Bowes AM, McCluskey J, Sim DF (1990a) 'Ethnic minorities and council housing in Glasgow' *New Community* **16** (4): 523–32

Bowes AM, McCluskey J, Sim DF (1990b) 'The changing nature of Glasgow's ethnic minority community' *Scott Geograph Mag* **106** (2): 99–107

Bowes AM, McCluskey J, Sim DF (1990c) 'Racism and harassment of Asians in Glasgow' *Ethnic Racial Stud* **13** (1): 71-91

Brah A (1992) 'Women of South Asian origin in Britain: issues and concerns' In: Braham P, Rattansi A and Skellington R *Racism and Antiracism: Inequalities, Opportunities and Policies*. Sage, London: pp64–78

Bryan D, Dadzie S and Scafe S (1985) *The Heart of the Race: Black Women's Lives in Britain*. Virago, London

Clifford J and Marcus G E (1986) *Writing Culture: the Poetics and Politics of Ethnography*. University of California, Berkeley

Cox J and Bostock S (eds) (1989) *Racial Discrimination in the Health Service*. Penrhos Publications, Newcastle-under-Lyme

Currer C (1986) 'Concepts of mental well and ill-being: the case of Pathan Mothers in Britain' In: Currer C, Stacey M (eds) *Concepts of Health, Illness and Disease: a Comparative Perspective*. Berg, Leamington Spa

Donovan J (1986) *We Don't Buy Sickness, It Just Comes*. Gower, Aldershot

Douglas J (1992) 'Black Women's health matters: putting black women on the research agenda' In: Roberts H (ed) *Women's Health Matters*. Routledge, London, pp33–46

Doyal L (1985) 'Women and the National Health Service: the carers and the careless' In: Lewin E and Oleson V (eds) *Women, Health and Healing: Towards a New Perspective*. Tavistock, London: pp236–39

Finch J 1984 '"It's great to have someone to talk to": the ethics and politics of interviewing women' In: Bell C and Roberts H (eds) *Social Researching: Politics, Problems, Practice*. Routledge and Kegan Paul, London: pp70–87

Froggatt K (1985) 'Tuberculosis: spatial and demographic incidence in Bradford 1980-82'. *J Epidemiol Comm Health* **39**: 20–26

Goel KM (1981) 'Asians and Rickets' *Lancet* **2**:: 405–406 and other articles

Greater Glasgow Health Board (1989) *Annual Report of the Director of Public Health*. GGHB, Glasgow

Greater Glasgow Health Board (1990) *Annual Report of the Director of Public Health*. GGHB, Glasgow

Greater Glasgow Health Board (1991–2) *Annual Report of the Director of Public Health*. GGHB, Glasgow

Health Committee (1991–2) Report on Maternity Services *House of Commons papers 29.1*

Howlett BC, Ahmad WIU, Murray R (1992) 'An exploration of white, Asian and Afro-Caribbean peoples' concepts of health and illness causation'. *New Community* **18** (2): 281–92

Kazi H (1986) 'The beginning of a debate long due: some observations on "Ethnocentrism and socialist-feminist theory"' *Feminist Rev* **22**: 87–91

Kitzinger S (1992) 'Birth and violence against women: generating hypothesis from women's accounts of unhappiness after childbirth' In: Roberts H (ed) *Women's Health Matters*. Routledge, London: pp63–80

Lawrence E (1982) 'In the abundance of water, the fool is thirsty: sociology and black "pathology"' In: Centre for Contemporary Cultural Studies. *The Empire Strikes Back: Race and Racism in 70s Britain*. Hutchinson, London: pp95–142

Martin E (1989) *The Woman in the Body: a Cultural Analysis of Reproduction* . Open University Press, Milton Keynes

Matheson LM, Dunnigan MG, Hole D, Gillis CR (1985) 'Incidence of colo-rectal, breast and lung cancer in a Scottish Asian population. *Health Bull* **43**: 245–9

McAvoy B (1990) 'Women's health' In: McAvoy BR, Donaldson LJ (eds) *Health Care for Asians*. Oxford University Press, Oxford: pp150–71

McAvoy BR, Raza R (1988) 'Asian women: (i) Contraceptive knowledge, attitudes and usage (ii) Contraceptive services and cervical cytology'. *Health Trends*. **20**: 11–17

McKie L, Gregory S, Garrett T, Bellerby I (1990). *Patterns of Take-Up and Attitudes Towards the Cervical Smear Test in the County of Cleveland*. North Tees Community Health Council, Stockton-on-Tees

Miles R (1989) *Racism*. Routledge, London

Oakley A (1980) *Women Confined: Towards a Sociology of Childbirth*. Martin Robertson, Oxford:

Oakley A (1981) 'Interviewing women: a contradiction in terms'. In: Roberts H (ed) *Doing Feminist Research*. Routledge and Kegan Paul, London: pp30–61

Opie A (1992) 'Qualitative research, appropriation of the "other" and empowerment'. *Feminist Rev* 40:52–69

Parmar P (1982) 'Gender, race and class: Asian women in resistance'. In: CCCS *The Empire Strikes Back: Race and Racism in 70s Britain*. Hutchison, London: pp236–75

Pearson M (1986) 'Racist notions of ethnicity and culture in health education. In: Rodmell S and Watt A, *The Politics of Health Education: Raising the Issues*. Routledge and Kegan Paul, London: pp38–56

Phoenix A (1988) 'Narrow definitions of culture: the case of early motherhood'. In: Westwood S and Bhachu P (eds), *Enterprising Women: Ethnicity, Economy and Gender Relations*. Routledge, London: pp153–76

Ramazanoglu C (1989a) *Feminism and the Contradictions of Oppression*. Routledge, London

Ramazanoglu C (1989b) 'Improving on sociology: the problems of taking a feminist standpoint'. *Sociol* **23**(3): 427–42

Ramazanoglu C (1990) *Methods of Working as a Research Team* (Women Risk and AIDS Project Paper 3). Tufnell Press, London

Rathwell T and Phillips D (eds) (1983) *Health, Race and Ethnicity*, Croom Helm, London

Roberts H (1985) *The Patient Patients: Women and their Doctors*. Pandora Press, London

Roberts H (1992) 'Answering back: the role of respondents in women's health research'. In: Roberts H (ed) *Women's Health Matters* Routledge, London: pp176–92

Rocheron Y (1988) 'The Asian Mother and Baby Campaign: the construction of ethnic minorities' health needs'. *Critical Social Policy* **8** 1: 4–23

Rocheron Y, Dickinson R, Khan S (1989) *The Evaluation of the Asian Mother and Baby Campaign: Synopsis*. Centre for Mass Communication Research, University of Leicester, Leicester:

Scott S (1992) 'Evaluation may change your life, but it won't solve all your problems'. In: Aggleton P, Young A, Moody D, Kapula M and Pye M (eds) *Does it Work? Perspectives on the Evaluation of HIV/AIDS Health Promotion*. Health Education Authority, London

Smith P (1991) *Ethnic Minorities in Scotland*. Scottish Office, Central Research Unit, Edinburgh

Stanway A, Stanway P (1984) *Choices in Childbirth*. Pan, London

Wardhaugh J (1990) *Asian Women and Housing: the Potential for Community action* Unpublished PhD thesis, University of Stirling

CHAPTER 5
MEN'S PERCEPTION of PREGNANCY

Vicki Taylor

The subject of pregnancy could feasibly be seen to fall neatly into the field of medical science. Antenatal care and the biological aspects of pregnancy tend to be firmly located in such traditions.

This study considers the experiences and different perceptions of pregnancy by exploring with a small group of men their experiences of their partner's pregnancy.

The decision to focus on men's feelings and experiences about pregnancy was based on a number of reasons. First, I was interested in and personally committed to the research question. As a woman who would eventually like to move towards parenthood, I had some personal interest and investment in the research question. I had begun to contemplate the implications of children for my own relationship hence the area of inquiry seemed to have relevance for me which is important since:

> ...no one is really interested in understanding something that is totally irrelevant for (her)himself and for the society in which (s)he lives. We are interested in something because of what it stirs up in us; because of our political commitment; because of our own personal history (Rowan and Reason, 1981).

Second, there appeared to be a dearth of health education literature concerning men's feelings. Health education in general (especially in areas related to pregnancy) does not focus on men's experiences and emotions; ostensibly there was a gap in provision. As Morgan acknowledges:

> We know more about wives and mothers than about husbands and fathers. (Morgan,1991,p94)

or about the process of becoming a father. Third, to legitimise the view that men have feelings and experiences in relation to issues which are often dismissed as women's matters seems to be of significance to both men and women. Many men are completely unprepared, both emotionally and intellectually, for the birth of their child(ren). In my own circle of friends, I was aware that most of the conversation amongst 'pregnant couples' was from the woman's position. Consequently, I felt strongly that a dialogue would benefit both women and men.

Images of pregnancy

As previously discussed (Taylor 1992) Graham's (1977) review of visual images of pregnancy in parentcraft literature illustrates how the introduction of images of men in antenatal literature served to reinforce the view that a woman could only fully attain motherhood providing her 'husband' was an active supportive partner. Pregnancy in the 1970s, Graham argues, was simultaneously portrayed as a period of health and a time of sickness, being both physiologically normal and emotionally stressful, at the same time natural and medically problematic. A decade later Meerabeau's (1987) discussion of the images of fatherhood expresses similar ambivalences, suggesting that little has changed.

A more recent analysis of depictions of pregnancy and parenthood in parentcraft literature (Dingwall, Tanaka and Minamikata (1991)) notes that contemporary official versions of parenthood emphasise parental choice and decision making rather than expert prescription. They observe that there are no assumptions that parents will be married and that men are portrayed as being as involved as women. However, from the review of the literature undertaken for this study, men's involvement continues to be portrayed in terms of the active supportive partner. Virtually all of the literature is devoted to motherhood and childcare. Most books relating to pregnancy present only a few pages or at most a chapter addressed to the 'expectant' father. Where men are addressed, they are not encouraged to consider their emotional needs (exceptions include Shapiro, 1987; Hearn, 1983; Bradman, 1985).

The predominant message given is that pregnancy is a stressful and emotional period for women and that men should aim to minimise this stress by adopting a supportive role.

Researching fatherhood

Recent developments in research on fatherhood have begun to challenge previous research which concentrated solely on mother-child relationships. Much of the impetus comes from the women's movement, where feminists have challenged the traditional notion which claimed that motherhood was the natural status for women. Richards (1982) explains that interview studies of women's experience of pregnancy and delivery have formed a prominent part of a wider interest in female reproductive experience and that theoretical perspectives have ranged from a generally feminist orientation (e.g. Oakley, 1979) to a concern about the effects of changing obstetric practice (e.g. Chard and Richards, 1977). There has been a shift in the literature in the last decade to include the experiences of men as well as women. Richards suggests that this shift parallels men's greater involvement in antenatal classes and hospital deliveries. However, he argues that the starting point for much of the research has been the growing dominance of medicine as the social institution that defines and controls the experience of pregnancy and birth for women. Similarly, much of the research on men has focused on their experience of the medical establishment and has rarely considered their emotions and feelings.

Less interest has been shown in the connections between men's feelings about their partner's pregnancy and delivery and other aspects of their own lives (Richards, 1982:61).

Men not only have to deal with their own confused feelings and uncertainties about their partner's pregnancy, but also face uncertainty and contradictory messages from those around them.

Developing the research question

In line with feminist criticisms I believe it is important to provide an embodied account of the research process (Harding,1989) . A number of influences affected my decision to focus on feelings and experiences in the way that I have done; these include an interest in reproductive issues and a belief in allowing individuals to have a say in matters which affect or relate to them.

I wanted this study to be a co-operative inquiry in stark contrast to the type of research I had been steered towards in my biological background and I wanted to explore an area which is often ignored or not acknowledged by Health Education. These concerns developed into an examination of men's experiences and feelings in relation to their partner's pregnancy.

The evolution of the research question was as follows. The first few months consisted of redefining the research question, thus supporting Fransella's thinking that

... the whole of the early part of a research project should be concerned with exploring, elaborating and almost certainly reformulating the research question. (Fransella, 1977:37)

I first became interested in men's feelings while focusing on a media case study where I had been interviewing women about their feelings and concerns in relation to abortion. While participating in this, I was consciously aware that I was ignoring men's feelings and concerns. Although I had specific reasons for choosing to focus exclusively on women I was uneasy about the situation. As my interviews progressed my concern to consider what men thought was strengthened. More significantly, the partners of some of the women I interviewed wanted to be involved, were eager to talk at length about many of the issues which had materialised during the interviews and wanted to discuss their own feelings in relation to abortion. There seemed to be a genuine interest and willingness to explore sensitive issues.

Questions which have to be asked about any piece of research include: what am I (the researcher) interested in; is the research useful, and to whom; is the research worthwhile and for whom? In a sensitive area further questions arise: might the research cause harm; would the research be beneficial; was it ethical; what would be feasible or realistic; to whom might I have access and how would the research be conducted? As these questions and further criteria were considered, the research question was modified and went through the transformations stated in Figure 1.

The question Why focus on men? still begs further exploration. I am conscious that, on the one hand, I could be accused of trivialising feminist positions. However, I do not think that the exclusion of men in such discussion is helpful. I would argue that as women we are more likely to see the connections between our experiences and the work arising out of the women's movement.

Men, on the other hand, have to work against the grain — their grain — in order to free their work from sexism, to take gender into account. (Morgan1991:95)

Morgan (1981) argues that the central requirement of a non-sexist methodology is that of always taking gender seriously and that, up until recently, 'taking gender into account' has usually meant taking women into account. As Roberts (1981) acknowledges, 'a non-sexist methodology should, in a literal sense, bring men back in'. This study conducted in 1987–8 takes men's experiences and feelings to be central and attempts to do so in a non-sexist manner.

Figure 1

What are men's feelings about abortion	May 1987
What are men's perceived needs in relation to abortion and how might they be met by Health Education	June 1987
How do gynaecologists' views concerning men's involvement in pregnancy counselling affect their practice	July 1987
What are men's counselling needs in relation to abortion; and what implications does this have for health education	Sept 1987
Is abortion a health education issue	Oct 1987
What are men's feelings about pregnancy and what are the implications for health education	Oct 1987
Pregnancy — a shared experience? An examination of men's feelings and experiences of a partner's pregnancy, implications for Health Education.	Nov 1987

By questioning and exploring the area of pregnancy from this perspective, I hope to influence the current role of health education and its emphasis on providing information for women (with the intention of bringing about behaviour change) to include men. My concern is to promote the view that men have emotions and feelings, and that it is healthy to acknowledge such feelings and probably beneficial to mental health — an issue which health education is only just beginning to address.

Methods: Methodological and practical issues

In searching for methods to explore men's feelings and experiences of pregnancy I was concerned to develop an approach which would capture and describe men's feelings and experiences. The methodology adopted required elements characteristic of a case study, while acknowledging and allowing maximal co-operation between myself and the men with whom I worked. In addition, I was concerned that the methodology chosen was compatible with my resolve to work in a non-sexist way.

There are a number of issues which remain unresolved within qualitative research methodology. Researchers using qualitative methods have often been confronted with questions of validity, bias and reliability in their research. Habermas (1971), in his proposal for a consensus theory of truth, argues that there is need for self-reflection which recognises 'its underlying technical interest' combined with verstehen — or understanding — to form critical-dialectical knowledge. Parlett (1981) appears to subscribe to a view which acknowledges the importance of consensus in relation to validity when he states 'that there is no absolute and agreed upon reality that has an objective truth' (1981:224). Rather, there are numerous different perspectives, many of which enjoy consensual validity. Such approaches resonate with feminist writers who have argued that it is important to examine the 'individual variety' of people's lives 'to learn from it before we try to generalise-since generalisations can so easily become the imposition of self and erasure of other' (Geiger 1986:334).

Feminist researchers have made concerns which others view as unproblematic central in their struggle with issues of power and control in the research process. These concerns include questions of power and control between researcher and researched, debates about the status of interview data, and questions concerning the production of 'objective' data and analysis which encompass issues of validity, reliability and bias. Feminist theorising has approached these issues even to the extent of questioning or rejecting the perspectives which generate such concerns or the notion of 'objectivity'(however this does not mean a rejection of the need to be critical, rigorous and accurate (Du Bois (1983)).

In the context of the research described here a few of the issues raised within this debate are particularly relevant. Firstly, rather than seeing the individuality of the researcher as a source of bias to be eliminated from the research some feminist methodologists have written of the importance of locating themselves within their work (Roberts (1981); McRobbie (1982); others suggest that this is something which should be evaluated and made visible within the data (Cornwell (1984); Morgan (1981); Oakley (1981); Harding (1987)). The researcher's values and theoretical stance will influence the choice of research question and the way in which data is selected. Therefore it is important that these aspects are made available in the research process. Feminist methodology insists that the researcher is located in the 'same critical plane as the overt subject matter' (Harding 1987:9).

As Stanley and Wise point out

'Whether we like it or not, researchers remain human beings, complete with all the usual assembly of feelings, failings and moods. And all of these things influence how we feel and understand what is going on. Our consciousness is always the medium through which the research occurs; there is no method or technique of doing research other than through the medium of the researcher' (Stanley & Wise1983:157).

Cain (1990) in her discussion of feminist standpoint epistemology considers issues of validity and accountability by discussing how the choice between 'science' and 'unscience' (or experience) can be overcome. She argues that knowledge produced from a standpoint must 'work' for those from whose standpoint it was produced. In addition, and perhaps more importantly, she argues that any theory derived from this data must explain both the researcher and the researched.

Feminist methodology also raises the question of the status of accounts given by those participating in the research process and how these are treated. Similar considerations have been discussed in 'New Paradigm' research which is grounded in a philosophy which values the interaction between the researcher and those researched and respects the contributions which can be made (Rowan and Reason (1981). This contribution may be strong in the sense that the subject is co-researcher and contributes to creative thinking at all stages. Or it may be weak, in the sense that the subject is thoroughly informed of the research propositions at all stages and is invited to assent or dissent. Rowan and Reason believe that New Paradigm research aims to minimise alienation and to maximise the potential for social change. At the level of consciousness a permanent change of ideology may be required of the researcher. Such aims were implicit in my research question and influenced my final choice of methodology, however the difficulty in accomplishing the abandonment of a hierarchical research relationship and achieving a more democratic research process was something which, on reflection, I was not fully prepared for.

I fully supported Stanley and Wise's claim that traditional research and research relationships often involved treating people as 'objects', 'there for the researcher to do research on'(1983:170) and their objections to such an approach but in practice this proved to be more complex. Morris and Gelsthorpe (1991) describe the difficulty of dismantling power differentials between female researchers and men who are the researched and the potential implications of this, however, in this study the difficulties encountered were more closely related to normative expectations of what constituted an interview.

Getting Started

In September 1987 I deliberated for some time on how I would contact men willing to participate in this study. It seemed a daunting task. Asking male friends whose partners were pregnant or had recently experienced becoming a father to be involved was discounted. I eventually went through the sequence of events depicted in Figure 2.

Figure 2: The research process and its network effect

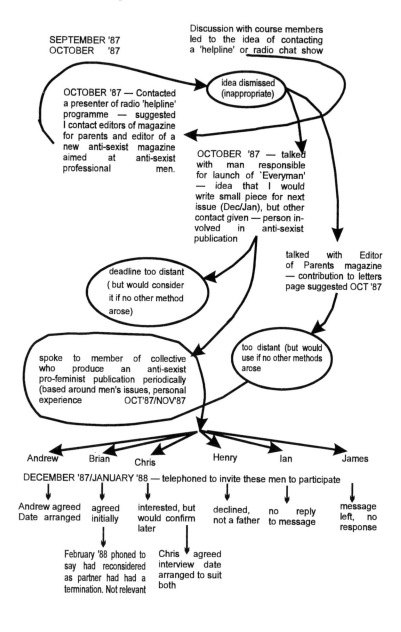

While working in Coventry as a Health Education Certificate Course tutor, I was presented with a golden opportunity when I was involved in a student health education practice assessment. The student was working with an antenatal group in the West Midlands which had been organised to include expectant fathers. The sequence of events arising from this situation are detailed in Figure 3.

Figure 3

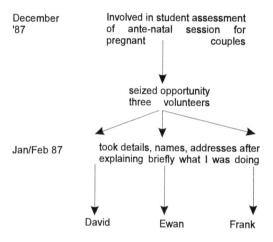

The aftermath of these events resulted in me interviewing a total of five men:two of whom had expressed a commitment to anti-sexism and collaborative childcare; three who may or may not have had such a commitment[1]. This selection procedure clearly has little to do with randomisation or selection according to fixed criteria. Of more importance was my concern to find men who were

---

1   *This information was volunteered by the men concerned*

sufficiently interested in the work to participate as fully as possible. I wanted to pursue men's experiences and feelings surrounding pregnancy; this seemed to be particularly relevant to those men who were about to become parents as well as to those who had already agreed to be involved. The men in the situations described here were probably somewhere along the spectrum towards the kind of emotional exploration that I was engaged in: they are not necessarily representative of parents and expectant fathers in general[2], but they were all involved (and still are), to a greater or lesser degree in their partner's pregnancy and subsequent childbirth.

The discussion of issues concerning men, pregnancy and emotion presented is based upon five interviews which varied in length from forty five minutes to two hours, in the participants' homes.

All of the interviews were informal and consisted of my probing and asking those interviewed how they felt about issues and concerns that they raised. I am aware that at times I directed the flow of the interview although I made a conscious effort not to intrude. By adopting this approach, I was attempting to develop what Massarik (1981) describes as a humanistic style of interview, encompassing characteristics such as acceptance, trust, a fundamental equality between interviewer and interviewee, a commitment to a search for joint understanding and an empathetic effort to enter the other person's world. However, it is more likely that in the course of this study I achieved the level of interview Massarik refers to as the 'depth interview'. In this style of interview, the interviewer wants to explore the views and perceptions of the interviewee in depth.

Each of the men who agreed to become part of the study was

---

2   *Clearly a number of men are not interested and those interviewed in this study are not typical*

given a written outline of the research process and it was emphasised that the focus of the research was to develop an understanding of the feelings and experiences they felt were important, how pregnancy had affected them and any other issues that they considered to be of significance. Each interview began with a recap of the letter I had sent explaining the nature of the interview which was followed by my saying 'over to you'. In this context the interview resembles a guided conversation, similar to everyday conversational practices, designed 'to elicit rich, detailed materials that can be used in qualitative analysis' (Lofland (1971:76). For this reason, no specific interview schedule was used to direct the interview. Instead, participants described what they had perceived to be important and occasionally responded to enquiries such as 'How did that make you feel?' Research of this kind is often criticised for valuing the particular and subjective experiences at the expense of scientific rigour. Its value is in yielding detailed, extensive data not usually achieved through conventional focused interviews. The major advantage of this method is the richness of material generated and the ability to reach issues and feelings which would otherwise be unavailable.

One of the difficulties this methodology poses is reflected in the complex nature of analysing the data provided. My approach was to dutifully transcribe all of the interview tapes and to categorise their contents. Each of the men interviewed was encouraged to be involved in this process, to check transcripts and to amend information relating to them as appropriate and also permitted a sharing of experience between researcher and researched. Each interview has been checked by the interviewee and the right to alter or amend information has been preserved. Throughout an attempt to preserve anonymity was emphasised and all participants were aware that they could withdraw from the research at any point (taking their data with them if they wished).

My intention throughout was to gain an understanding of those feelings and experiences they considered important, how pregnancy had affected them and any other issues that they considered to be of significance. Ostensibly, in pursuing this area of inquiry I had made a number of assumptions: I had assumed that men can experience and relate to pregnancy in some way, that men have emotions, experiences and feelings concerning their partner's pregnancy and that they would be conscious of these. Collaborative research assumes that the researcher and researched have the same commitments and motivation to the inquiry. Most of the men interviewed saw themselves as the subjects of the research and their expectations of what constituted research meant that they did not wish to be such active participants.

It is important to take into account the relative status and power of the researcher and the researched. Oakley argues (1981) that conventional interview techniques frequently treat the researched as objects to be made sense of through the researcher's analysis. Silverman refers to this as the 'asymmetry of interactional rights' (1985:167). A conscious attempt was made to conduct the research as a shared study, but as Graham has noted, 'the researcher's goal is always to gather information,' hence there is always a danger of manipulating relationships to that end. Acknowledging unease about certain aspects of the research role is not necessarily a drawback. On the contrary, it heightened my awareness of the burdens of such intrusion, however collaborative in spirit, into people's lives and the responsibilities such involvement carries.

Each of the men interviewed had particular views concerning me — those based in the West Midlands may have seen me as somehow involved or connected with ante-natal education which may have directed the information given to me[3]. Written

---

3   One of the men interviewed commented that he thought I was a health
      visitor, it is possible that the other two who volunteered to take part in this
      study also saw me as being connected to the antenatal class they were
      attending when they volunteered despite my explanation that I was doing this

information, together with telephone conversations would have enabled them to develop a picture of the kind of person I was, which could have influenced the interviews. Similarly, the fact that I was a female could have been significant. On the one hand, the men I interviewed may have revealed less to me than if I had been a male, while on the other hand I may have learned more. I do not know, but think it more likely that as a consequence of the socialisation process which acknowledges that it is acceptable to value interpersonal skills in a woman, I was able to establish rapport and work from a more personal basis. My approach throughout was to develop a friendly, open relationship based on mutual respect as far as possible. Each interview varied tremendously and I am aware that a more comfortable, co-operative, intimate relationship was established in some interviews. This ultimately affected the personal risks I was prepared to take, in addition to the outcomes of the interview. Where there was a common interest, or it was apparent that we agreed on many issues, I am conscious that the length of our interaction was greatly extended. Furthermore, my commitment to co-operative inquiry meant that the style of interviewing was possibly more accessible to those men who had been involved in men's groups and had expressed a commitment to anti-sexist work.

This, then, is the context in which this study took place. I have outlined the purpose of the study and sketched in some of the background details. This material has been submitted in an attempt to acknowledge the assumptions, perspectives, experiences and feelings that informed this study. In the next section I would like to introduce and provide a portrait of each of the men based on their self-descriptions, my perceptions and the information they divulged during the course of the interviews.

It may be significant that none of the men interviewed found

---

as a research project for my MSc

describing themselves an easy task and in all cases they commented on the difficulty of self-description. Finally, I have included their responses, where appropriate, to my request to reflect on how they felt about the interview.

I was concerned to use the interviewees' own words wherever possible in order to minimise the possibility of mis-representation; consequently all of the experiences and feelings I relate are unique.

Andrew

Andrew lives in a large Victorian house in London in the Inner City. My encounter with Andrew was one Sunday afternoon in January when he answered his door with a sleeping child in his arms.

I introduced myself and was made welcome. The interview between myself and Andrew took place in the kitchen over numerous cups of coffee. We seemed to develop a rapport and responded to each other well, which clearly influenced the interview. He describes himself in the following way:

I'm 37, white, male. I work as a counsellor part-time at a post-adoption centre. I've got two children, 2 and 4, both boys. I'm living with my wife who also works part-time. We've been together about thirteen years; a long time. I've lived in London for most of my life. I currently live in Hackney, where we've lived for at least fourteen years. As I mentioned in the interview, I was adopted, and that's had a lot of bearing on my response to being a parent. I think I'm probably much more preoccupied with the whole issue of parenting partly because I was adopted. I don't really know what to say about myself without going on at great length.

On completion of this interview, I had a lengthy discussion with Andrew about the mechanisms for increasing collaborative childcare — an issue I personally was interested in. Issues such as employment, alternative work options and the politics of the current status of women and men in relation to childcare were touched upon. Additionally, I offered advice concerning sources of funding for workshops for men regarding parenting — recognising and making explicit the potential for contribution and support from Health Education for such a venture.

Reflections on the interview experience — six months on

Reflecting on the interview, I recall feeling at ease and interested in Andrew's situation. As the interview progressed I found myself identifying with the way in which Andrew and Sally had approached parenthood. The interview was very informal and relaxed and was aided by the thought and consideration Andrew had given it. Andrew's reflections on the experience refer to the preparation he made prior to the interview. He explained that having the chance to think about his views beforehand was useful and more beneficial than if he had been interviewed cold. He concluded by saying that it was an enjoyable experience: a view I would endorse.

Chris

I first spoke to Chris in December and finally interviewed him in March. Chris lives in a flat in an Inner City area in London. The interview took place while Chris was caring for his son, James, in the kitchen. He comments that the interview situation seemed somewhat unreal in his reflections on the interview.

My own interview with you I also found slightly unreal, in that James was sitting on my lap at the time — I was talking partly about him, which he was aware of, but he couldn't understand the detail. He was co-operative and attentive but also competing for attention. Still, it worked OK.

My own feelings concerning the interview would agree with this, however there was no intrusion.

I think that we developed a rapport very quickly (possibly helped by the numerous telephone conversations prior to meeting) consequently I was relaxed and interested in what Chris had to say.

My interviewing technique had developed considerably by this stage and I had internalised areas which seemed to be important. Consequently, I felt more confident and at ease with the interview situation. Additionally, Chris had interviewed others himself which I suspect helped our situation.

Chris expressed difficulty describing himself initially, but offers us the following sketch:

I'm Chris, born in 1947, which makes me 41. I've been in a relation with Val, who's James' mother for about ten years or possibly more. James is now 2, we're actually planning at the moment, we're trying to start a second kid. We're not married, we live together, and we don't necessarily intend to live together but we might do, we might not. We both work part-time, look after James part-time.

My job is public-transport campaigning, I used to be a town-hall planner, transport planner.

I was brought up in the suburbs of Surrey in a conventional nuclear family with one brother.

I've travelled a fair bit abroad to a lot of different countries, some with Val and some not.

I don't know what to say really, I don't know what sort of things it's worth saying.

[Well, how would you describe yourself?]

What, mentally?

[Whatever you think is important.]

I don't know, I find it really difficult to do. I'm sort of a, bit of a sort of individualist, by which I mean although I do get involved in collective projects, I do quite like doing things on my own, so having a kid is one of the things I've obviously done with somebody else and I like doing things together, but I also like being an individual. So actually having a kid is a bit of a conflict between the two sides of myself a) being in a group and doing things together and b) wanting to do things on my own and the two things are a little bit of a conflict, so I end up having a slightly split life as a result of having a kid.

Doing things on my own tends to be done in the midnight hours when I'm not responsible for the group project which is helping look after James. The decision to have a kid is a big one too, it's a conflict between the individual in myself and your desire to do things with other people and I'm aware of it. I sometimes explore it by writing things but usually I skip over it. I've written quite a few things on various things, I want to write more, I've got aspirations as a writer. I've been involved in one, maybe two men's groups at various times, neither of them very long-lasting, one about a year or so. I didn't get incredibly emotionally involved in either of them. The first one was intellectually more interesting, the second one was with a group of friends and that was difficult. The first one was led by somebody who's relatively experienced and now going on to do more things like that.

He chose to run a therapy group, and the second one was neither consciousness-raising nor therapy, because we were friends and had different relationships with one another, we actually never got down to brass tacks in the group, so it didn't work basically. I've also dabbled in co-counselling more recently and there's a parent's group that I've been along to once, and I might do that again soon. We did at one time have a group of fathers as well. There was about four or five of us and that was quite interesting although it folded. Now we see each other as individuals either with or without the kids. Now I do get involved in mutual aid with other people and their children, joint child-care and that's really good, excellent. I don't know if you want me to answer

*what sort of person am I, I don't know if that's relevant, and I
don't know if I'm qualified to say.*

[Whatever you think.]

*As a kid I was always very shy. I was the shy and brainy one of
the family as opposed to my brother, who was the extrovert and
naughty and physical and practical. I've probably come towards
the centre of those attributes. I enjoy young James and I find it
very frustrating as well.*

[Thanks, that's great.]

At the end of the interview, Chris and I talked for a considerable
time about male politics and the current position. James was also
the subject of some discussion.

Reflections on the interview experience-four months on.

Reflecting on the interview, I found it fascinating and was interested
in Chris's situation. At times it drifted, but this was necessary to
allow Chris to consider and present his thoughts. I felt at ease with
the interview situation and confident enough to avoid becoming
directive, although I probed and asked questions during the course
of the interview. Chris's comments are positive, helpful and
generally support my perception of the experience:

As to how I felt about the interview experience.

*I think it went pretty well. You obviously got me to talk- so your
approach of letting me do the talking worked. I notice from
reading the transcript that you had a list of basic brief questions,
but they were experienced by me as your just asking how I felt
about (a), (b) or (c) and then simply listening while I responded.
It worked, because you were non-judgmental (something that
rarely happens in ordinary conversation) and were `interested'.*

*Such interviews tend to be slightly surreal, in that the interviewer
appears to suspend judgement.*

So the interviewee is occasionally thinking 'what's her emotional response to what I've just said?' But since your guard didn't slip and you always remained 'interested but neutral', I presumably felt safe enough to carry on talking.

As I've found when I interview people, the interviewee actually rather likes the interview experience, because it allows them to explore some of their own emotional undergrowth — a relatively rare opportunity to do so at some length.

David

David lives with his wife Elaine and their child in a modern house in the West Midlands. The interview took place on a Sunday evening in February. Elaine and the baby were out at relatives. The interview began fairly quickly having established and agreed its aims. I liked David and seemed to be able to communicate effectively with him and the interview itself was very relaxed -two factors which may have influenced the nature of the 'data'.

David is an engineer, studying part-time for a BSc in Mechanical Engineering with an optimistic view of life. He describes himself after some deliberation in the following way:

Well, my name is David. I'm 27 years of age and I've been married 6 years in August. I'm a fairly athletic person, I'm fairly shy really in situations where there are new groups getting together.

I'm not very outgoing until I get to know people. I'm not a particularly career-minded sort of person, I'm not a particularly emotional sort of person either. I don't very often show love and care to people. I'd regard myself as mediocre intelligence, average run-of-the-mill sort of thing.

Probably I've got a fiery temper and can sometimes quite easily show that, it's the red hair.

Is there anything else?

[It's up to you]

I sometimes take on more things than I can cope with, I like to get involved socially in things.

Sometimes it doesn't go down very well with Elaine, I suppose sometimes I can be a bit selfish.

Sometimes I think of myself and other times I can probably be a bit over-powering in thinking of other people. That's about it really.

[Right, thanks very much.]

Okay.

[Yes, that's lovely, thanks very much.]

Reflections on the interview experience — 5 months on:

On reviewing this interview I was surprised at the warmth it revivified for me. David's warm personality and enthusiasm for life are implicit in his accounts. In response to my request to comment on the interview experience, David says that:

The interview experience was quite soul-searching. To be fair I found I had to look critically at my actions, especially where I may have been selfish and it can be equally as hard to be modest.

He suggests that :

It may have been useful for Elaine to have been consulted for her opinion on what I have said. I do feel however that I have tried to be unbiased and tried to relay the many aspects and changes.

and that

It may, in hindsight, have been advantageous to conduct three interviews, i.e. three months into the pregnancy, six months and three months after. The reasoning behind this is that I found it difficult to relate emotions and changes which took place six months previous.

He explains that in retrospect he is not

.&... too happy with my reply about the changes I felt at the time between knowing about the pregnancy and towards the end, i.e.. the middle three months.

and has since thought about this and can only conclude that

&... this must have been a period of change where the thoughts of responsibility and character changes actually took place.

I will consider these points further in the next section.

Ewan

Ewan lives in a modern house in the West Midlands. I arrived slightly later than arranged, one wet evening in March. Immediately I was made welcome by Ewan and his wife Jane. Ewan described their relationship as a relatively equal one and compared it with his parents whose marriage was very much more one-sided.

The climate in which I've been brought up has made me believe in far more of a two-sided marriage where the partnership is more of an equal one, and hopefully it is. Both of us have no set jobs, like you do the gardening and you do the washing-up and the washing.

The fact that it may in some ways come out like that because of the amount of work that I do and the amount of time Jane's at home is just it's happened like that. Normally, if a job needs doing we go off and do it, so I end up doing the washing-up, and the cooking, the cleaning, washing clothes or whatever. The way that both of us operate is probably more equal except for her because there is no way I can provide the same as Jane does, I just ain't got the equipment.

The interview was carried out in the lounge accompanied by numerous cups of coffee, chocolate biscuits, two dogs, Jane and Kate. Jane occasionally contributed to the interview, reinforcing or clarifying what Ewan had said (although these comments were not clear enough to be transcribed and have been omitted from the transcripts) but did not detract from Ewan's comments.

I was relaxed and felt that an understanding between us was developed with ease.

Ewan is an electronics technician and is studying part-time. He has a wonderful sense of humour and frequently uses analogies to describe his perceptions — neither of which are adequately captured on paper.

He describes being involved in his wife's labour in the following way:

It was much better to be actually in there and discover it more at first-hand. Sort of is this it or is this not it? In some ways it must be like paratroopers feel like before they go over enemy territory, it's like being in the aircraft before you jump out, and you don't really know what's going to happen down there, but there's no way you can back out of it.

Ewan found it particularly difficult to represent himself. In his words:

It's difficult, part of me feels I shouldn't quote my academic achievements because it's a form of elitism.

[Well choose what you feel is important.]

It's not looking at yourself too hard in some ways, in other ways being quite proud of things you've achieved, but in other ways angry at your mental and physical shortcomings because of society's pressure to be an achiever. Wherever you've got to there's always going to be somebody that's bigger than you, that's achieved more than you, that's done more than you, is cleverer than you, and not wanting to blow your own trumpet in such a way that you appear pompous. You can describe yourself as ugly, thick and uncouth.

[Having said all that, how would you describe yourself?]

Do you regard the age as important as regards to the views expressed because of the way that the different age groups express their feeling on new fatherhood? A man in his thirties would perhaps regard fatherhood in a slightly different way than a teenager, that's unmarried and scared.

[Where do you put yourself?]

In some ways I could describe myself as a 26 year old electronics technician of average intelligence, with an abiding interest in sport. Lives in an average house with an average wife. I'm trying to be classless about it as well. Probably basically that.

I stayed for almost an hour after completing the interview, talking with both Jane and Ewan, which was an enjoyable experience. I learnt from Ewan that he felt he had not really discussed his feelings or emotions although a reading of the transcript suggests otherwise.

Reflections on the interview experience — 4 months on:

I recall the interest and enthusiasm generated by the interview when reflecting on the experience.

Ewan's letter to me seems to mirror this. He states:

The interview was quite an interesting experience because it made me focus on the pregnancy and my feelings towards the whole process.

It would appear that this was one of the first times that Ewan had seriously considered such feelings.

He describes it as an 'odd' experience, but also as a 'useful' one.

The interview also made me take stock of my life at that particular time and the feelings towards the most important people in it to me. It was also an odd experience to be put on the spot because I was not used to expressing my personal inner feelings to someone I had met only briefly before but it was useful in the fact that I had to confront and relive some of the most anxious moments of my life.

Frank

Frank and Sharon live in a modern detached house in the West Midlands with their child. They are both graduates and have lived in London as well as the Midlands.

The interview was arranged for a Sunday afternoon by telephone and confirmed in writing— although I suspect I had made some error in the address since I was aware that the expectations of the interview and the interview itself did not match closely. On a technical level it is significant that during the interview the tape-recorder stopped: this meant that some repetition occurred in the interview as we tried to remember what had been covered previously. These factors may well have affected the interview.

I was made welcome and the interview began in the lounge although we moved almost immediately to the dining room. Sharon was periodically present during the interview and I suspect this influenced its content.

I learned that Frank and Sharon had carefully planned their child and had been fortunate enough to be very organised prior to the birth. Frank's job was important to him and involved a considerable amount of travelling. He describes himself in the following way.

[So would you mind describing yourself?]

Nearly 31, a Midlander. I've lived in London for a while and worked in various parts of the country.

I travel a lot around the UK. I live in a detached house and have been married five years in August this year. My wife, I met her in a hotel in Sutton Coldfield, we've both lived in London for a while.

I would say I was, in terms of class group, I would say I was in the so-called professional classes rather than the working class, middle-class or whatever. I classify myself as the professional class, not particularly sporty, useful around the house, decorating, things like that. I find it easy to investigate and work out the best plans, I'm not the type to stick my head in the sand and hope things go OK. I'd say fairly sociable, I like a quiet weekend though because I have to see a lot of people during the week.

[What else?]

This is our second house, we're mortgaged up to the hilt, like everyone else, taxed to the hilt like everyone else and fairly aspiring for various things. A planner I would say, I think that's important from your point of view to understand that. I like where we live and wouldn't want to change. We're not really into holidays. I can't think of anything else unless you've got any questions about me.

Once the tape recorder was switched off we continued talking for about thirty minutes. Sharon was interested to know more about my research question and I explained that I was concerned to find out more about men's feelings and experiences of pregnancy and that it was for that reason I had not used a formal interview schedule. I was interested in Frank's feelings not mine. Her response was illuminating — she suggested that it was unlikely that Frank would discuss his emotions with me whatever method was chosen — this is likely to be the case for many men.

During this discussion Frank questioned me about the framework within which I was placing this study, drawing on his own experience and perceived necessity for agenda-setting. This was also reflected during the interview when asked:

[Are there any other questions you think I should be asking?]

*It's very difficult for me to understand whether you've missed
out a whole range of questions because I can't see how I fit in the
sample.*

[Well really what I was getting at was were there any particular
things that you expected me to ask or you felt are important that I
haven't picked up? I've tried to leave it fairly open-ended so that
the men I interview can actually tell me what they think is
important, but at the same time I've also picked up on certain
things. I've got some ideas, but I don't want them to influence what
comes out.]

*Well, if you're looking at the care of the child or helping a future
father is how the project is going to be used. If it's helping the
father then it's probably been covered, I mean the key thing is to
be prepared. If it's to do with the welfare of the child thereafter
then we haven't covered it at all.*

[No, it's to do with how men feel about their partner's pregnancy,
and their experiences of that.]

*Yes, I suppose it's to do with whether it's planned or not planned.
There's probably more shock in an unexpected one where your
wife came home and said she was pregnant, your reactions would
probably be quite different. The only question I think that could
have been talked about in more depth is the social standing of
the father or his job.*

Reflections on the interview experience — 5 months on:

Looking back on this interview I remember feeling anxious that
my tape-recorder stopped during the interview and feeling that I
had not sufficiently clarified with Frank what I was endeavouring
to do. Consequently I asked more questions and directed the flow
of this interview more than I did in others. Re-reading the transcript
there appear to be sections where Frank discusses his emotions and
feelings, but generally he talks about practical issues and offers

advice for others. For me, the interview raises issues which may be considered problematic and need to be resolved when undertaking research of this nature.

Frank would have liked to have corrected the grammatical and syntactical presentation of this interview but time-constraints did not allow this.

Main findings

At this stage it is customary to reflect upon exactly what the research means, to explore what might be learned and to consider the implications of the issues raised. In this section I will look at some issues which arise in all of the interviews and then consider their implications for health education. One issue identified in the interviews relates to the way in which a partner's pregnancy is perceived. In all of the interviews a partner's pregnancy is referred to as an abstract or remote experience for the men concerned and their alienation from the physiological process is commented upon. Other points emerging from the data are associated with change, transition and the resultant conflicts arising from the moment of becoming a father: adapting to new work patterns; different friendship patterns; changing relationships and lifestyles; altered self-image and the development of new personal politics. A further prevalent metaphor suggests that the experience of a partner's pregnancy can be liberating for men in that doors to a whole new, previously unknown world are opened. These issues can be represented by the following diagram (Figure 4) and will be explored further in the next section.

The remainder of this chapter elaborates and expands on each of these representations and some implications and recommendations for health education are drawn out.

Figure 4 Three prevalent themes arising from interviewing men about their feelings and experiences in relation to pregnancy

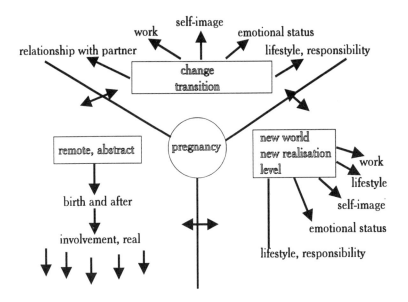

Pregnancy as an abstraction

In most cultures pregnancy is seen to be a woman's concern (Lamb 1986). Childbirth is often a period for women alone, men's personal feelings and needs often ignored. Subtle pressure is exerted upon men to stay in the traditional role as supporters to the pregnant women. Subsequently, men often do not find the support and encouragement they need to negotiate the transition to parenthood. Because men are remote from the physiological process of pregnancy, it can seem intangible for some time. It is, therefore, understandable that many men feel distanced and alienated from the pregnancy. Each 'expectant' father encounters this experience differently; some are more involved, while others remain detached. This is not altogether surprising since in our patriarchal[4] society men have been encouraged to remain on the periphery of childbirth.

All of the men interviewed in this study expressed feelings of alienation and had some difficulty relating to the pregnancy, feeling excluded by the fact that it was enclosed in their partner's body as expressed in the following extracts:

...because you're not going through the thing at first hand, you can lend your support, but it's a bit like being at a football match spectating because there's all this going on somewhere else and you're there watching it. You feel like your role is to be there as a support, but no matter how much support you give you can't go through the same thing as the women are [Ewan].

I can remember feeling, the emotional period wasn't so much during the pregnancy and the birth, it was after the birth when I could feel things, when James was actually there. Instead of me trying to relate to someone else's physiology, somebody else's emotions...I wasn't pregnant, I didn't breast-feed and I didn't give birth, it wasn't actually connected to me...before that [the birth] it was all very academic [Chris].

It cannot be over-emphasised that the experience is unique for all expectant fathers, but all men are physically remote from the process. Men are actively encouraged to participate in pregnancy, childbirth and childcare and, at the same time, physiologically forced to retain a peripheral role.

Antenatal classes were cited by the men interviewed as a way of becoming more involved in their partner's pregnancy. However, many men are reluctant to attend because they feel such classes are not relevant to them-often they are correct. One of the men interviewed expresses his frustration at being encouraged to be

---

4   *I am using `patriarchal' in the way that Hearn describes it: Hearn (1983), Birth and Afterbirth: A Materialist Account, Achilles Heel, London, p8, p55*

involved and then feeling ignored when he attempted to find out more:

It felt annoying because you felt you could ask her things, but you didn't really get any answers to some of the things you were asking. They were saying about asking questions all the time, and you could get some answers out of them, but it was like for them they took all these antenatal classes and they went through the set things every time, and then if you put them out of their stride by asking them something they weren't really used to, they tried to go in a different direction so they didn't have to answer it [Ewan].

Another recalls how, during the pregnancy, he went to active birth classes with his partner, an experience which he describes as enjoyable but somewhat remote:

Although I enjoyed that and it certainly helped a lot in thinking about what was to be done, I think I felt increasingly, and a lot of men said it too, I can only think about after the birth, I couldn't really think about the pregnancy. I kept thinking about what would happen when the baby was born...I remember feeling quite shy, I suppose everyone else was quite shy...it was very much a female thing...it was all done on the woman's territory... [Andrew].

It was clear from the interviews that emotional conceptualisation of pregnancy takes time to become a reality. It was not until there was some substantial evidence of pregnancy that these men were able to relate, albeit superficially, to their partner's pregnancy. As the development of the child progresses each of the men interviewed was able to feel more involved:

Well, it got more real. I suppose the thing that made it much more real was the scan. Once you see the scan it brings it much more home because up till then there's the gradual getting the `bump' and all the rest of it, but you could just be sort of eating too well, and then you see the thing with the four limbs and the heart beating, moving round on the scan. That's the beginning of the *realisation [Ewan].*

The first effect was when I saw the ultrasound, that I'd recommend to any future father. It's fantastic, the technology to be able to see the baby there. That was the first point I realised something fantastic was happening, there was a baby growing there, waving its hands...I could have sat there all day watching it. I was telling the lady doing the ultrasound, `This is fantastic. I wouldn't miss this for the world!' [Frank.]

For those men who saw ultrasound scans and were present at the birth, pregnancy developed from a concept to an intensely emotive, real experience.

Pregnancy as transition

Oakley (1979) demonstrated the profound emotional shock posed by motherhood for many women. However, since there is little public recognition of `expectant' fathers and their emotional needs, preparation for parenthood can be seen as more complex for men than for women. As Seel (1987) observes:

Pregnancy is a time of great change and uncertainty for many men, perhaps made worse by the fact that society as a whole does not acknowledge the powerful effect it can have on them...

Added to this, there is overwhelming evidence that boys and girls are treated differently from birth and that, in the process of learning gender differences, certain qualities are suppressed in men (gentleness, tenderness, emotional expression, caring) while being reinforced in women (Mead (1949); Rosenberg and Sutton-Smith (1972); Chodorow (1978); Wellings (1984)). Other characteristics associated with men (competitiveness, aggression, success, dominance) are suppressed in women. When boys learn to be men they must reject unmanly characteristics such as vulnerability and emotional spontaneity. The disadvantages for women of such cultural ordination have been documented by feminist writers

(Delphy (1984) and, more recently, the disadvantages for men have gained some interest (Seidler (1988)). Pregnancy was seen by all of the men interviewed as a transitory period. One describes the experience as a 'happy period' and as something which was 'fun'. For others, it is a worrying and emotionally significant phase bringing with it a number of stresses, strains and unresolved contradictions. Areas which seemed to be of particular importance (at least to men in this study) centred on newly acquired ambivalent attitudes towards paid employment and the impact of new responsibilities on current lifestyles and their self concept. Each of these areas were interrelated to form a complex web of tangled emotions.

The responses of the men interviewed indicate that their experience of pregnancy is powerful but remote. The notion that pregnancy represents the end of freedom and a dramatic change in lifestyle was raised by all of the men to a greater or lesser degree but of greater significance was their alienation from it. Relationship fears were expressed during the interviews. In some cases, men feel that their relationship with their partner assumes a secondary position compared with their partner's relationship with their child. Other studies corroborate this. Shapiro (1987) suggests that this fear of losing the relationship plays a significant role in late-pregnancy affairs. A tenth of the men he interviewed acknowledged having an affair in the last phase of their wife's pregnancy and cited feelings of rejection as the main motivational factor. Clearly, men's ability to confront such fears is important for their relationships.

Feelings of responsibility are heightened as a consequence of becoming a parent. Prior to the birth of a first child, the majority of couples are both in paid, full-time employment. As pregnancy progresses, concerns about finance are common. Where a woman is giving up work, the expectant father is often acutely aware that he will be the primary financial provider, a legitimate concern in today's economic climate. Two of the men interviewed in this study (Ewan and David) were in the situation where their wives had been made redundant, thus they were now solely responsible for generating income. Their situation appears to have fostered ambivalent attitudes to paid employment. They talk about, on the one hand, the need to take their job more seriously, while on the other hand, their desire to be at home more:

This thing about being the breadwinner suddenly fell on my shoulders you know...my job was going to be more important now than it had been in the past. I used to work a fair bit of overtime, but that didn't matter anymore to me. I realised my responsibility was being with Elaine in case anything happened, and I made a conscious effort to be at home more... [David].

Unsurprisingly, attitudes towards job security and future prospects became more of an issue than they were previously:

It's all linked in because you feel now that you are the sole provider that you've got to be in some ways better than you were before because of the position of responsibility that you now hold...I think it's affected my attitudes to work in the way that before I would have been more ready to look round for another job that was less secure in order to perhaps gain more finance, whereas now I look at the job that I'm presently in and I think well, it's reasonably good money and it's reasonably secure... [David].

Relatively few men resolve the dilemma of the competing demands of careers and of families, even fewer adopt part-time or job-share options.

Two more of the men interviewed (Andrew and Chris) had made a commitment to be involved in collaborative childcare with their partners. In accordance with this, it was necessary for them to negotiate new employment patterns after the birth of their children, changing from full-time to part-time paid employment. For Andrew, this also involved finding a different employer. Both talked of the difficulties involved in `going against the grain'. Those that opt for paid employment on either a part-time or job-share basis as Andrew and Chris have done, become acutely aware that the way in which society is structured is unsupportive. Fein (1974:12) summarises the dilemmas faced:

Society provides little support — whether financial or emotional — for men who want to spend regular time caring for young children. Economic pressures and the press toward a successful career often force a man to choose between his work life and his family life, an anguishing choice that some men are refusing to make.

Although this was written almost twenty years ago it is notable that the situation remains unchanged, reinforced by the lack of childcare and other family support.

Pregnancy as confrontation and liberation

Responses to the interviews indicate that, for these men, this period in their life was the first time they had considered themselves in any depth. Their considerations ranged from: reconsidering their personal politics and re-evaluating themselves; rekindling an interest in their own origins; to agonising over and accepting their own inevitable infallibility and insignificance in the order of things.

Pregnancy forced them to reassess and reformulate their personal politics. As a result of becoming a parent, one of the men recalls being re-politicised and ʻbecoming more committed to the world at large', another describes how his personal politics have become less distanced, more related to habitual issues which touch people's lives on a daily basis:

Things like whether a local health centre closes. Most people, most political activists don't know there's a local health centre, so how can they know whether it's closing or not, what do they know about the effect that has on the people that go there? So actually having a kid does change your politics...male politics is a bit of a laugh actually, half the time...child benefit is a major political issue, but how many blokes could you get to show an interest in it whatsoever? [Chris].

Of all the considerations prompted by pregnancy, none is so profound or confrontational as the realisation of the fragility of humanity. Shapiro (1987: 27) suggests that pregnancy and birth serve to highlight the reality of death which is often hidden in our culture:

Since death is so much avoided and kept from daily awareness, while birth is expected to be such a happy event, most expectant fathers were surprised by their feelings about the fragility of human existence. As they begin to anticipate the birth of a child, however, men begin to ponder such issues.

Chris reports how he felt forced to consider his own mortality for the first time and how glad he feels to have had this opportunity:

...it makes you face up to certain philosophical and biological realities which before you can avoid thinking about and are encouraged to avoid thinking about. People are afraid of death, for instance, whereas when you have a kid you're aware that death is a possibility at any moment and birth, birth and death, these sort of great biological possibilities become much more real when you actually have to experience them. Everybody's expendable and a lot of things are a matter of chance [Chris].

Others describe an increased sense of connection to their own familial roots and report feeling much more closely attached to their own fathers. This was particularly pronounced at the birth of their children as familial characteristics were much in evidence, creating concerns such as `Will I be a good father?' and `Will I make a better job than my parents?'

One of the men interviewed describes how his partner's pregnancy enabled him to consider, for the first time, his feelings about being adopted as a child:

I was adopted when I was a baby and I was brought up by my adoptive parents, I mean that's okay, but I think for me there was this particular dimension about the birth. Two things happened to me, one is it reawakened my interest in my birth family which had sort of lain dormant, and I thought I must really find out more about my birth family and I went and got my birth certificate and the adoption agency records which you're entitled to do and I hadn't done that before...and then it dawned on me that the child that was going to be born would be my only blood relative that I'd ever met, so I think for me probably more than other men, though I think everybody brings to childbirth some very deep and powerful feelings, they were very much centred on my own origins and where I had come from [Andrew].

Richman (1982) states that pregnancy provides men with an important opportunity for emotional involvement. More recently, Seidler (1988) charts the dilemmas and contradictions faced by men in acknowledging their emotions and needs. Nevertheless, all of the men in this study comment on how differently they felt about themselves as a consequence of their partner's pregnancy, and put succinctly by Ewan, '*you know that from the point of birth you're never going to be the same again*'.

Discussion: implications for health education

The men who agreed to participate in this study had one important factor in common: they were all actively involved in their partner's pregnancy. These fathers may not be representative but as McKee and O'Brien (1982) suggest:

Finding out about fathers and campaigning for a change in their situation may have important consequences for women and men, for we share with Poste the hope that `when men share housework and childcare with women, important mechanisms of patriarchy are threatened'.

The patriarchal assumption that men are the chief breadwinners and women their economic dependants is reinforced by the laws on employment, social security and taxation which define economic dependence as women's normal status. Despite significant increases in cohabitation, divorce and one parent families, which appear to undermine the traditional patterns of family life, family law and welfare benefit systems continue to endorse the position that men are providers and women are dependent wives and mothers. New and David (1986) observe that `...*men can push prams, women can be bank managers, but as the exceptions multiply, the rule itself is untouched*'.

Research undertaken for the Equal Opportunities Commission by Bell, McKee and Priestley (1983) and more recently by Hollerman and Clarke (1992), and Delphy and Leonard (1992) concludes that the structural arrangements in our society do not facilitate a more active role for men as parents. Although an increasing number of couples are in a position to rearrange their work commitments so that they may take shared responsibility for childcare, they still represent a minority. Despite the concepts of paternity leave and joint childcare slowly gaining acceptance, there are still strong peer pressures (in spite of high levels of unemployment) for men to seek paid employment and, in the UK, to work long hours. Paradoxically, the climate for the possibility of other arrangements is increasingly acknowledged but social attitudes which continue to reinforce the status quo. The challenges for health education are immense and wide ranging, dependent upon the philosophical perspective adopted. A commonly agreed key element of health education is information giving. The information and advice related to areas such as antenatal care, relationships and childcare should aim to include and portray men in roles other than the traditional breadwinning, supportive role.

In times of increasing male unemployment, health educators have an opportunity to reflect the fact that more men are becoming involved with children (although this may be by default rather than design). Care should be taken to actively portray men as `emotional beings' who are able and willing to participate in their partner's pregnancy and subsequent childcare at both an affective and practical level. The representation of men publicly caring for children and participating in domains traditionally allocated to women can all work to influence societal norms and social attitudes.

Currently, 'parenting' preparation (generally referred to as childcare) is taken up by girls — although there are some exceptions — reinforcing stereotypical sex roles. On a broader level, health education activities, and in particular those relating to relationships, should aim to challenge those stereotypes which work against men expressing their emotions and feelings. More initiatives resembling the Family Planning Association's Men Too campaign, Channel 4's About Men programmes and Albany Video's Becoming a Parent should be encouraged and supported.[5] In addition, health educators should continue to work to influence publications to reflect such challenges. The Health Education Authority and District Health Education Units are uniquely placed to promote and undertake such work since:

> *...those who make decisions on what does and what does not get published have an active role in shaping a discipline or area and this raises legitimate cause for concern for those attempting to work in ways which challenge mainstream orthodoxies (Spender, 1981).*

Co-existing with initiatives already described is the need for Friere's (1972) concept of 'conscientisation' or awareness building. The first task is to enable people to believe in themselves. Health education of this sort inevitably becomes process-orientated, based on the principle that people learn as a group and from one another. It is a process through which members of the group(s) develop an

---

5   See *Wellings (1986), Men Too: A retrospective view of the FPA's male responsibility campaign, FPA, London; Morrison P, Eardley T and Humphries N (1983), About Men, Channel 4; White J and Morrison P (Directors) (1986), Becoming a Father, Albany Video Enterprises, London*

understanding of each other's perceptions which, in turn, causes individuals to question their own ways of life and brings the realisation that there are alternatives. Involvement is action. Co-operative, non-hierarchical approaches to parenting from within the community should be supported and encouraged. Many of these initiatives involve raising awareness, challenging the status quo and are implicitly concerned with societal change.

Health education activities which subscribe to and campaign for the notion of parental leave, lobbying and working with multidisciplinary bodies, including industry, trade unions and local government should be actively supported.

Job share schemes and part-time employment are more prevalent than even a few years ago, but relatively few men are represented. The goal should be to enable parents, whatever sex, to opt for job share schemes and part-time work and to obtain parental leave, thus challenging some of the structural and economic forces upholding patriarchy. Furthering the adoption of parental leave; establishing job share schemes for both women and men; viewing men as fathers as well as workers and women as workers as well as mothers are important challenges for health education. In Bradman's (1985:261) words:

> *I'm talking about creating a world in which there is a new fatherhood as part of a new way of looking at both men and women. We have to accept the fact that there are differences and go beyond mere acceptance into a celebration of those differences. We also have to realise that just as there is a part of every women which has been denied up to now — her more `masculine' part, her independence and assertiveness — so the `feminine' side of men has been repressed and distorted. What we must do is create a society in which both men and women can develop every area of their personality and lives, as far as is possible and as much as they want to.*

The following recommendations are offered as a framework for action:

- identify and consider those issues that men and women collectively identify as significant to pregnancy, childbirth and childcare

- act upon community based and environmental factors which affect the health of men and women as identified in this context

- unify and integrate 'top-down' and 'grass roots' initiatives

- address, re-assess and change the concepts of 'father' and 'mother' to 'parenthood' at the level of ideas

- support changes in social relations by monitoring differentiation of service provision, prejudice and discrimination

- work to secure a more genuine participatory form of health education which inevitably will embody a participatory politics of reproduction

- (re-)educate those who control access to and provision of resources in order to reduce 'sexist' resource allocation

PostScript

Within sociology interview data is often considered problematic. A dilemma exists, namely whether interviews can be seen as straightforward accounts of an external reality or whether they create and report upon their own structures. From an interactionist framework, interviews are merely one type of interaction between participants, social events which are accomplished by the researcher and researched in a specific, situated, context. Any consideration of the interview situation, according to this perspective must take into account 'the latent identities that the participants invoke and attribute to one another' (Hammersley and Atkinson (1983):119) when considering the meaning and significance of the data generated. As a consequence Hammersley and Atkinson (1983):119) question the extent to which data obtained during the course of an interview can be generalised to other situations. This argument coincides with a concern with what Goffman (1959) termed 'presentation of self' whereby people engage in 'presentation management' in an attempt to control how others perceive them. As Shaffir (1991:130) notes individuals may 'choose to emphasise one of several selves that they sense is most appropriate' given the interview situation. Extending this further, Silverman has described interview statements as providing 'access to a set of moral realities firmly located in the cultural world' (1985:16). The conclusion Silverman draws from this is of the need to analyse interviews as embedded 'situated' practices. This does not mean however that the content of what is said in an interview situation is of no sociological interest.

References

Bell C, McKee L, Priestley K (1983) *Fathers, Childbirth and Work*. Equal Opportunities Commission, Manchester

Bradman T (1985) *The Essential Father*. Unwin Paperbacks, London

Cain M (1990) 'Realist philosophy and standpoint epistemologies of feminist criminology as a successor science'. In: Gelsthorpe L, Morris A (eds) *Feminist Perspectives in Criminology*. Open University Press, Buckingham

Cain M, Finch J (1981) Towards a rehabilitation of data. In: Abrams P *Practice and Progress in British Sociology*

Chard T, Richards MPM eds (1977) *Benefits and Hazards of the New Obstetrics*. Heinemann, London

Cornwell J (1984) *Hard-earned Lives: Accounts of Health and Illness from East London*. Tavistock, London.

Chodorow N (1978) *The Reproduction of Mothering: Psychoanalysis and the Sociology of Gender*. University of California Press, Berkeley

Delphy C (1984) *Close to Home: A Materialist Analysis of Women's Oppression*. Hutchinson, London

Delphy C, Leonard D (1992) *Familiar Exploitation. A New Analysis of Marriage in Contemporary Western Societies*. Polity Press, London.

Dingwall R, Tanaka H, Minamikata S (1991). Images of Parenthood in the United Kingdom and Japan. *Sociol* 25 3: 423–46

DuBois B (1983) 'Passionate scholarship: notes on values, knowing and method in feminist social science'. In: Bowles G, Duelli Klein R (eds) *Theories of Women's Studies*. Routledge and Kegan Paul, London.

Fein RA (1974) Men and Young Children. In: Pleck JH, Sawyer J eds, *Men and Masculinity*. Prentice-Hall, New Jersey: 54–62

Fransella F (1977) *Personal Constructs Psychology*. Academic Press, London

Friere P (1972). *Pedagogy of the Oppressed*. Penguin, Harmondsworth

Geiger S (1986) 'Women's Life Histories: Method and Content' Signs. *J Women Culture Soc* 11: 334–51.

Goffman E (1959) *Forms of Talk*. Blackwell, Oxford

Graham H (1977) Images of Pregnancy in Antenatal Literature. In: Dingwall R, Heath C, Reid M, Stacey M eds, *Health Care and Health Knowledge*. Croom Helm, London

Habermas J (1971) *Knowledge and Human Interests*. Beacon, Boston, Mass.

Hammersley M, Atkinson P (1983) *Ethnography: Principles in Practice*. Routledge, London

Harding S (1987) *Feminism and Methodology*. Open University, Milton Keynes

Hearn J (1983). *Birth and Afterbirth: A Materialist Account*. Achilles Heel, London

Hollerman S, Clarke K (1992) *Parents, Employment Rights and Childcare: The Costs and Benefits of Improved Provision*. Equal Opportunities Commission, Manchester

Lamb ME (ed) (1987) *The Father's Role : Cross-Cultural Perspectives*. LEA *by Vicki Taylor*

London

Lofland (1971)

McKee L, O'Brien M eds (1982). *The Father Figure*. Tavistock, London: 23

McRobbie A (1982) 'The politics of feminist research: between the talk, text and action'. *Fem Rev* 12: 46–57

Mead M (1949). *Male and Female: A Study of the Sexes in a Changing World*. Morrow & Co, New York

Meerabeau E (1987). Images of Fatherhood in Antenatal Literature. *Health Visitor* 60: 79–80

Morgan D (1981). Men, masculinity and the process of sociological inquiry. In: Roberts H ed, *Doing Feminist Research*. Routledge and Kegan Paul, London

Morris A, Gelsthorpe L (1991) 'Feminist Perspectives in Criminology: Transforming and Transgressing'. *Women Crim Just* 2 (2): 3–26

New C, David M (1986) *For the Children's Sake*. Penguin, London: 43

Oakley A (1979) *Becoming a Mother*. Martin Robertson, Oxford

Oakley A (1981) 'Interviewing Women: A Contradiction in Terms'. In: Roberts H (ed) *Doing Feminist Research*. Routledge, London

Parke RD (1981) *Fathering*. Fontana Paperbacks, Glasgow: 22

Parlett M (1981) Illuminative Evaluation. In: Rowan P, Reason J (eds) *Human Inquiry : A Sourcebook of New Paradigm Research*. John Wiley & Sons, Chichester

Richman J (1982) Men's Experiences of Pregnancy and Childbirth. In: McKee L, O'Brien M eds, *The Father Figure*. Tavistock, London

Richards MPM (1982) How should we approach the study of fathers? In: McKee L, O'Brien M eds, *The Father Figure*. Tavistock, London: 57–71

Roberts H (1981) *Doing Feminist Research*. Routledge and Kegan Paul, London: 4

Rosenberg BG, Sutton-Smith B (1972) *Sex and Identity*. Holt, Rinehart & Wilson, New York

Rowan J, Reason P eds (1981) *Human Inquiry: A Sourcebook of New*

Paradigm Research. John Wiley & Sons, Chichester: 134

Seel R (1987) *The Uncertain Father: Exploring Modern Fatherhood*. Gateway Books, Bath: 39

Seidler V (1988) Fathering, Authority and Masculinity. In: Chapman R, Rutherford J eds, *Male Order: Unwrapping Masculinity*. Lawrence & Wishart, London

Shaffir W, Stebbins R (1991) *Experiencing Fieldwork: An Inside View of Qualitative Research*. Sage, London

Shapiro JL (1987) *When Men are Pregnant: Needs and Concerns of Expectant Fathers*. Impact, California

Silverman D (1985) *Qualitative Methodology and Sociology*. Gower, Aldershot: 167.

Spender D (1981) The Gatekeepers: A Feminist Critique of Academic Publishing. In: Roberts H ed, *Doing Feminist Research*. Routledge and Kegan Paul, London: 87

Stanley & Wise (1983)

Taylor VJ (1992) Pregnancy:A shared experience? *J Adv Health Nurs Care* 2(2): 59–78

Taylor VJ (1986) *Pregnancy:A shared experience? Co-operative enquiry into men's experiences and feelings about pregnancy*. Unpublished M.Sc. thesis, Centre for Educational Studies, Kings College, University of London.

Wellings K (1984) *Men in Relationships: A Selected and Annotated Bibliography of Recent Books and Journal Articles*. Family Planning Association, London.

CHAPTER 6
WOMEN'S EXPERIENCE of ANTENATAL CARE in TOWER HAMLETS

Ruth Cochrane

Abstract

Antenatal care has been criticised by consumers, and eliciting their opinions about the service is important if practice is to improve. A survey was conducted among 955 women receiving antenatal care in Tower Hamlets in East London, where several options for antenatal care exist. Women's expectations and actual experiences are described with reference to their type of antenatal care. Those having antenatal care in the community were more likely to be satisfied with their care than those having hospital based or shared care. Obstetric outcomes were either comparable between these three groups or slightly improved in the community based women. Community based antenatal care is safe, acceptable to women and should where possible be enhanced.

Introduction

Surveys addressing the consumer's opinion of antenatal clinics have been unanimous in their criticism of antenatal care (Garcia, 1982; Reid and McIlwaine, 1980; Taylor, 1986). The joyful anticipation usually associated with pregnancy is frequently dissipated by the clinic's anonymity and apparently inexplicable routines, a point illustrated by this old but unfortunately still pertinent extract:

`They just looked at my card and gave me a number — two

thousand and something. It was a case of take your place in the queue. But you don't feel with the first baby just one of the crowd — you feel you're number one. You have to realise you're just a number to them here' (Comaroff, 1977).

There is also an impression that the users of the service are not acknowledged as having an opinion, nor indeed any right to one:

`I said well what about the X-rays. And he said what X-rays. And I said, look I've had four X-rays and an ultrasound test supposedly to see whether I'm going to have a Caesarean or not. Don't worry about that my dear, we'll worry about that. Like I'm a real idiot, and he couldn't possibly discuss me with me. And he breezed off (Oakley, 1979).*

Reason for the study

A study commencing in 1989 of attitudes towards antenatal care in Tower Hamlets was timely since the maternity services there were entering a period of change with centralisation of deliveries in one unit and impending National Health Service reforms. Different forms of antenatal care, including community based care in which women receive all their antenatal care in local surgeries, exist in Tower Hamlets. The establishment of community based care has been shown to increase women's satisfaction with the service (Williams *et al*, 1989; Zander *et al*, 1978) with, in some cases, improvement in the obstetric outcome (McKee, 1982). Therefore, two obstetricians, a consultant and a research fellow planned to study women's experiences of antenatal care in the context of the type of care they received. The project was funded by Womanschoice, a charity supporting research into choice in maternity care. The charitable grant paid for the researcher's salary and for the stationery and computer discs required by the study.

Environmental and social background

Tower Hamlets is an area of cultural diversity and mixed fortunes. As well as the indigenous East Londoners, it is home to comparatively affluent young people who commute the short distance to the City, and a large number of people from various ethnic minorities. By far the largest of these is the Bengali community. Most of the older Tower Hamlets Bengalis originated in villages in rural Bangladesh and came to London seeking work, intending to return home as rich men. When it became clear that to return home would be unfeasible, wives and other family members were brought to London (Carey and Shukur, 1985). There is now a growing population of second generation immigrants in the area. Other ethnic groups such as Afro-Caribbean, Vietnamese, Chinese and Somalis are also well represented. Whilst some women from ethnic minorities are represented in the study sample, non-English speakers were not included since financial constraints prevented the use of interpreters.

The borough is a deprived area with a paucity of affordable private housing. The majority of residents live in cramped council accommodation, a source of animosity as described by Widgery (1991):

> *'the sense of neighbourhood, of overlapping families and the close proximity of work, pub and play characteristic of the old East End courts and terraces is turned into its opposite, a resentful proximity'.*

Local service provision at time of study

The borough has one hospital maternity unit at the Royal London Hospital in Whitechapel, where the vast majority of the borough's deliveries occur. There are hospital antenatal clinics here and at the Royal London at Mile End one mile away. Antenatal care is also carried out in general practitioners' surgeries and community midwives' clinics.

Most women have traditional 'shared care' with their general practitioner (GP) and the hospital clinic. Women deemed to be at high risk during pregnancy (e.g. diabetics) have all their care at the hospital by obstetricians and their junior staff. Women whose GPs do not undertake maternity care may also have hospital based care, attending hospital clinics staffed by obstetricians and hospital midwives, or may have all their care at a local community midwives' clinics after an initial consultant booking clinic visit.

One of the Tower Hamlets obstetricians has practised community based antenatal care since 1982. This involves women attending their GP's surgery for all their community antenatal care, where they are seen by either their GP or a community midwife. The surgeries are visited monthly by the obstetrician who sees all those who have just booked and anyone felt to be at high risk. This system, based on that initiated in Lambeth, provides specialist expertise to women registered in participating surgeries in a convenient and familiar setting. It also encourages professional autonomy amongst the doctors and midwives involved. Almost all the community based women will subsequently deliver in hospital but this may be the only time they visit the hospital.

Formulation of research question and design

Women's attitudes towards antenatal care and whether and how these attitudes differed according to the type of care they received formed the basis of the research question. This was to try to assess women's views about the local antenatal service when this service was undergoing a period of change. A scientific approach to this would have involved a randomised control trial with women booking for antenatal care being randomised to receive hospital care, shared care or community based care, and being questioned about their experiences in an impartial manner by a researcher blinded to the type of care they had received. In Tower Hamlets, these three types of care were already well established and to randomise women who would have been expecting one type of care to receive another would almost certainly have caused problems. For example, women who had formerly had a particular type of care, and liked it, may have been anxious about risking a change, and those who disliked the idea of one type of care may have worried about not being able to choose something different. Therefore, the study was designed to address a population already receiving care rather than randomising women due to receive care.

It was timely to enquire about women's preferences for antenatal care with a view to being able to inform women about their options and, hopefully, enhance the service. At the time of the study, the maternity services in Tower Hamlets were undergoing change as all the hospital deliveries were centralised at the Royal London Hospital at Whitechapel, having previously taken place at the Royal London at Mile End as well. Antenatal clinics still continued at Mile End as well as at Whitechapel, and community based antenatal clinics, a feature of the borough since 1982, were flourishing.

To question women about their experience of antenatal care after they had experienced it would have been a simple method of discovering women's preferences in the context of their prior expectations. This is a problem of women being satisfied with a system of care because it was the only one of which they had any experience, leading them to assume that it was more satisfactory than any other - a form of conservatism described by Porter and MacIntyre (1984). By asking about what women expected of care beforehand and then asking afterwards about their actual experience one could decide whether or not women were satisfied with their care because it had lived up to or exceeded their expectations.

Expectations may be formed and influenced by a variety of factors such as the attitudes of friends and family members, viewpoints expressed in the media and so on. Some women may have high expectations of the service and be disappointed by the reality they experience, whereas others will have low expectations and be pleased by whatever they receive. Thus, in this study, women's experiences of antenatal care have been examined in terms of what they actually received and how satisfied they were, given their prior expectations.

The original intention of the study was to include all women resident in Tower Hamlets booking for antenatal care over the course of a year. An attempt was made early on to include Bangladeshi women. It was hoped that the maternity aides who act as interpreters and advocates for the women in the hospital clinics would be able to help in the administration of the questionnaires. Whilst the maternity aides were as helpful as they could be, many real problems arose in trying to include women from this, the largest of the borough's ethnic minorities. The sheer weight of numbers combined with the lack of committed interpreting help, owing to the financial constraints of the study, made addressing all the Bangladeshi women impossible. The maternity aides were busy in the clinic with their normal work and often did not have time to do any `extra' interpreting. There was also a problem, one which bedevils any multilingual health service, with deciding on suitable interpreters. Family members would sometimes volunteer to speak on behalf of women but this was unsatisfactory since the answers they gave might not have been a reliable translation of the women's views but rather an exposition of their own. Unfortunately, those relatives likely to be the most fluent in English, such as husbands and sons, were the least suitable interpreters; husbands tended to express their own ideas rather than allow their wives to speak for themselves, and sons, especially youngsters, were embarrassed about or ignorant of the details of pregnancy.

The most difficult problem with trying to include the Bangladeshi women and the one that, finally, led to abandoning the attempt to include all the non-English speaking women in the study was the cultural gap. Even when a committed interpreter was found on a trial basis, she found it difficult to complete the questionnaires since many of the women did not understand the attitudinal questions. For them, the concept of choice in health care was unheard of: indeed, there is apparently no word for 'choice' in Sylheti, the dialect spoken by most of the Bangladeshis in Tower Hamlets. To describe feelings towards or criticisms of the maternity service would have been impossible for these women.

The result of highlighting these problems has been to improve the facilities somewhat for non-English speakers. A local service called Language Line was set up to allow a three-way conversation between the carer, patient and interpreter over a special telephone link. Initially, the service employed only Bengali, Hindi and Urdu speakers but it was hoped to include other languages in future. Another result was that a Sylheti version of the antenatal study was undertaken, administered by a Bangladeshi health worker.

Method and sampling

The plan was to perform a population study of all English-speaking women resident in Tower Hamlets over the course of a year to assess their experience of and attitudes towards the antenatal care they received. The questionnaires used by Reid *et al* (1983) in Glasgow in their comparison of hospital and peripheral antenatal clinics were used as a basis for the Tower Hamlets questionnaires. The Glasgow group had gone on to ascertain how their peripheral antenatal clinics related to the guidelines drawn up by the Royal College of Obstetricians and Gynaecologists (Williams *et al*, 1989) using the same questionnaires. It had been hoped that the later Glasgow study and the Tower Hamlets study would have been contemporaneous to allow comparisons.

Questionnaires

The structured questionnaires used in the study were modified from those used by Reid *et al* (1983) in their study of community based antenatal care in Glasgow. The questions were adapted by the consultant obstetrician supervising the study and by the research fellow who then administered the questionnaires to be appropriate for Tower Hamlets and for the particular interests of the study.

The antenatal questionnaires collected demographic information and also asked women to discuss their expectations of the antenatal services. Aspects of care considered in particular were the provision of reassurance and emotional support, having one's questions answered and procedures explained, receiving expert care, the provision of privacy for examinations, information on baby care, being able to see the same personnel at each visit and being able to see a woman doctor if one wished to do so. Questions were included about standard aspects of antenatal care such as taking blood pressure and palpating the abdomen. Other questions examined the more humane components of care such as receiving reassurance and seeing the same member of staff at each clinic visit. The postnatal questionnaires enquired about women's actual experience of care.

Examples of antenatal questions

- When you first booked with your GP, what choice were you given about where you could go for antenatal care?

- What choice were you given about where to have your baby?

- Do you think you have been given enough information about your tests?

Examples of postnatal questions

- Where did you go for your antenatal check-ups?

- What did you think of the clinics you attended?

- Where would you prefer to go for antenatal care?

The pilot study

Prior to undertaking the main study, a pilot study was performed. The antenatal questionnaire was piloted on 20 women in the waiting room of the Mile End antenatal clinic. The intention was to see how long on average the questionnaire took to administer and to identify any difficult or ambiguous questions. Once these women had been interviewed, three main conclusions were drawn. Firstly, each questionnaire took between five and fifteen minutes to administer, depending on how much extra information women wished to convey. Secondly, questions concerning women's knowledge of antenatal tests had to be rephrased on the basis of the pilot information. The original question had been 'which blood tests have you had?' to which the answer was invariably 'all of them', although very few women could describe what 'all of them' meant. The question subsequently became 'do you know the reason for any of your blood tests?' to which the majority of women answered 'no'. Those who did know the reason for some of the blood tests could then elaborate.

Thirdly, a question concerning whether or not a woman perceived the family income as adequate for their needs was omitted after the pilot study since all women answered 'yes', presumably because of the pride and independent spirit of the indigenous East End population, when for many the answer clearly should have been 'no'. It was less embarrassing for all concerned simply to enquire about occupation and deduce the income source from this.

The postnatal questionnaire was piloted among 20 women on one of the postnatal wards at the Royal London Hospital. These interviews took between 10 and 20 minutes to administer, again depending on how much more information women wanted give. Following this none of the questions were altered but the order of some of the questions was changed so that the flow from one to another was smoother.

The pilot interviews proved how willing women were to answer questions about their care. For many, the first questionnaire helped to pass the time while waiting to see the doctor or midwife. Following the pilot study and the ensuing revision of the questionnaires, the study proper began. It addressed women who booked for antenatal care between July 1st 1989 and June 30th 1990.

Logistic problems

Bearing in mind that this was intended to be a population study, there were several difficulties to surmount. Access was granted to five out of the eight hospital antenatal clinics each week, since only three out of the five consultants had given permission for women to be interviewed in their clinics. One of those refusing felt that as a large proportion of his patients had special pregnancy-related problems such as diabetes, they should not be included in the study. The reason for the other refusal is unknown. In addition, many of the Tower Hamlets antenatal clinics took place at the same time each week; Tuesday afternoon was a favourite time for appointments both in the hospital and in the community. Attempting to cover all the women seen in these clinics inevitably meant missing some of them.

Some women received all their care in the community; some attended the hospital clinic only once or twice and would be seen in the community for the rest of the pregnancy. In each case, it was not always a simple matter to see them straight after their booking visit and arrangements would have to be made to see them at their next community visit. This exercise would not always be efficient since there may not have been many others at the same clinic who were due to be interviewed and a special journey might result in only a small number being added to the total included.

One tactic for solving the problem of meeting women who

only visited the hospital once antenatally, if at all, was to conduct some of the interviews in local GPs' surgeries. Before embarking on these interviews, a letter was sent to all local GPs who undertook antenatal care to explain the nature of the study and to ask permission for some of the interviews to be conducted during their clinics. Each was provided with a tear-off slip which the doctor could sign and send back saying whether or not he or she objected to the idea. Almost 90% of those canvassed replied and none had any objection.

A plan was made of the location of the local practices and the times of their antenatal clinics. Inevitably, there were many clashes, with some times being very popular. On the other hand, a sizeable number of the GPs did not have an antenatal clinic per se but saw pregnant women during the course of their normal surgeries. These practices were not visited as a special trip would have wasted time if only one woman was interviewed and the timing would have been difficult to arrange during a busy surgery. Those practices that were visited were the ones with a scheduled antenatal clinic in which several women were seen in each session. Sixteen of the local surgeries fulfilled these criteria.

As far as the postnatal interviews were concerned, some women left hospital within a few hours of the birth and a very small number had home confinements. These, therefore, missed the interview.

A combination of the logistical problems of several different locations and the number of women involved meant that with one interviewer inevitably women were missed. Thus, once the interviews had started and it became clear that the study would not be of a total population, it was decided to interview as many women as possible.

Sample

In all 955 women (53% of the eligible total) were interviewed antenatally. Primigravidae (women expecting their first baby) formed 50% of the sample; 92% of the women were married or in a stable relationship, 83% were aged between 20 and 34 and 74% were in social class 3B to 5. The women interviewed were representative of the total of 1796 Tower Hamlets English-speaking residents who booked during the study period. There were no significant differences between the study women and the missed women in terms of support status, past history of intrauterine growth retardation or overall age, although there was a significant difference in the linear trend of age (p = 0.02).[1] There was a small but significant difference in the proportion of women who smoked (30.7% of the study women smoked compared with 26.1% of the missed women; p = 0.03) which is difficult to explain but probably unimportant except perhaps in terms of subsequent birthweight. There were significantly more primigravidae in the study population (39.2% compared with 30.5% of the missed women; p = 0.03). This is no doubt because of the preponderance of multiparae amongst women booking for community based care rather than hospital care and the former were more likely to be missed.

Postnatal interviews were conducted on 657 of the 955 women. Those missing left hospital soon after delivery, before the interviewer's morning visits to the ward. Obstetric data were collected from all but 23 of the 955 women (21 moved out of the area prior to delivery and two, unfortunately, had second trimester miscarriages).

One of the antenatal clinics not visited for the study was one in which there was a high concentration of high risk women, especially diabetics. These high risk hospital based women were not

---

1   *This calculation was performed using a series of chi-squared tests of significance, in which the number of cases in different descriptive categories are compared and analysed in relation to their **expected** and **actual** values*

included in the study. Women receiving hospital based antenatal care in this study did so because their GPs did not provide antenatal care. These women were not at high obstetric risk in comparison with those receiving shared care or community based care.

Conduct of research

Timing of interviews

The antenatal interviews were planned to take place after the initial booking visit by the midwife, so that tests and procedures would have been explained but before the women had become familiar with the clinic system. In terms of gestation, therefore, they took place between 16 and 24 weeks. Late bookers (i.e. after 28 weeks) were not included. The postnatal interviews were planned to take place while women were still in hospital following the delivery. Most were carried out on the first or second postpartum day.

Place of interviews

Interviews in the antenatal clinic at Whitechapel were carried out either in a small room adjacent to the waiting area or, if sufficient privacy could be assured and the small room was already being used, in the waiting area itself. Interviews at Mile End were also carried out in the waiting area. Both were large enough to ensure that the conversation was not overheard. This was important since some of the answers, particularly those concerning past obstetric history, could be deemed confidential. Interviews at community based clinics were carried out in small rooms set aside on the day of the clinic for the purpose. Each interview was carried out in the same way regardless of location, and the answers received were written straight on to a specially designed computer coding form.

Coding

Prior to commencing the interviews, some consideration had been given to the range of possible answers and these had been precoded with a number for each response to speed the transition from response to data entry. With practice, the correct number could be written directly on to the coding form as soon as the response was given and only with uncommon answers was there recourse to the master sheet later. This direct coding was done with both the antenatal and postnatal questionnaires and saved both time and paper.

Collation and analysis

The data entry was organised in such a way that the variables were in a logical order in relation to the coding form. Depending on the answer given, the cursor would either go straight on to the next variable or, if necessary, skip answers filling in figures meaning ' not applicable' and going on to the next variable in the sequence. Computer files were backed up regularly on to floppy discs and copies made of all the coding forms. The copies were stored separately from the originals.

Given the large number of women interviewed for the study, it was important to be able to keep track of them in a way that allowed rapid access to basic information along with a reliable method of storage. Details of each subject in the study were kept on an Agenda electronic organiser (Microwriter Systems PLC, 1988). This compact machine proved extremely useful not only for storage and rapid recall of information but also because of its word-processing facility. Names, hospital and study numbers and the expected dates of delivery for each subject were filed and could be called up instantaneously. Details relating to each subject could be edited and updated allowing progress to be checked (e.g. by adding D for 'done' after the second interview was carried out).

Lists could be produced, in alphabetical order if required of, say, all the women in the study due to deliver in a particular month. The expertise gained by using this tool has thus had several benefits in terms of the study.

Data were analysed using the computer statistics package Statistics Package for Social Sciences (SPSS) (Norusis, 1986) and using logistic regression analysis[2] with the Biomedical Data Program (BMDP) (Dixon, 1990).

Cross-tabulation and chi-squared tests were used, with p values of 0.05 or less considered statistically significant.[3] The analysis was first performed using SPSS-PC and further analysis to allow for confounding and explanatory variables used BMDP having first excluded non-significant variables. In this way, each outcome variable was examined using stepwise logistic regression as recommended by Bracken (1989).

The advantage of logistic regression over simple chi-squared tests appears when more than one variable is included in the statistical model. Simple chi-squared tests can say whether a variable is seen to have an effect on an outcome, but this may be due to its relationship was a real causal factor (for example, smoking and low social class). By introducing several variables into a logistic regression model, one can investigate the effects of variables on the outcome when taking into account other measured causative factors. By doing this in a stepwise manner, the computer selects only the relevant factors.

Tables can be constructed for each outcome under

---

2   *Logistic regression analysis is a statistical method for estimating the combined effect of different variables on different outcomes*

3   *The p-value refers to the likelihood or a `probability' of the effect being studied occurring by chance, i.e. that two factors (say smoking and low birthweight) are not causally related. The smaller the p-value, the greater the probability that the effect did not happen by chance*

consideration showing the numbers of subjects in each category, the odds ratio describing the odds of the outcome occurring to those women in one group as opposed to another, the 95% confidence intervals[4] and the p-value for each variable. Various computer software packages are available which will create tables or present results in a more graphical form with pie-charts, histograms and so on.

Results

Expectations of the service

Generally speaking, the women of Tower Hamlets have very high expectations of the antenatal services. Over 90% expected reassurance and emotional support, to have their questions answered and procedures explained to them. Almost 90% expected privacy and to have care from experts. Three-quarters expected to be able to see a woman doctor if they so wished and half expected to see the same person at each visit. Over 60% expected to be given information about baby care at the clinic.

There were some variations in expectations related to schooling, parity and fluency in English. Better educated women had more realistic expectations than less well educated women about receiving expert care (83% vs 91%; p = 0.01) and being able to

---

4   *Confidence intervals and odds ratios*
    Odds ratios are multipliers of the baseline odds so, for example, if the odds ratio for two groups is 2.5 then the odds of whatever it is being studied are 2.5 times higher in the study group than in the baseline group. Odds ratios are estimates of the real effects of different factors and when we take a sample we introduce sampling errors which make these estimates imprecise. Confidence intervals allow for this and give a range of likely values within which we are 95% certain that the real effect lies.

see a woman doctor (74% vs 91%; p = 0.01). Interestingly, there were no significant differences in expectations with relation to parity except regarding baby care information, with parous women less likely to expect this than nulliparous women (57% vs 71%; p = 0.0006). Women for whom English was not their first language were more likely than native English speakers to expect expert care (98% vs 88%; p = 0.02), women doctors (96% vs 75%; p = 0.0006) and to see the same person each time (75% vs 47%; p = 0.00005).

Perceived importance of aspects of care

Women were asked whether they felt particular aspects of antenatal care were important or not. Over 95% of women thought reassurance, having their questions answered and procedures explained and receiving expert care were important features of the clinic. Privacy was important for 85%, 77% wanted to see the same person each time and receive information on baby care, but less than half (48%) thought being able to see a woman doctor was important.

Actual experience of care

Around 75% felt they regularly received reassurance, answers to questions and understandable explanations, expert care and privacy. Less than half regularly saw a woman doctor and less than a quarter received information on baby care. Less than 10% saw the same person at each visit.

Comparisons between what women expected from the service and what they actually got revealed shortfalls in every aspect of care. Experience as a whole never lived up to expectations. This was especially the case with baby care information (62% expected this, 22% received it), being able to see a woman doctor if required (76% expected this, 50% regularly saw a woman doctor) and being able to see the same person at each visit (50% expected this but only 8% saw the same one or two staff members each time).

The impression is similar when looking at the factors women deemed important and the proportion of women actually receiving them, as again there were shortfalls for each aspect of care examined. The most striking differences between what women deemed important and what they actually received were with respect to baby care information (77% thought this important but only 22% received it at the clinic) and seeing the same personnel each time (77% thought this important but it was only a reality for 8%).

An analysis of the data was performed dividing women according to the type of antenatal care they received, i.e. hospital only, shared care and community based. Women who had community based antenatal care were more likely to see less personnel during their antenatal care than those attending hospital. Those seeing only one or two staff members comprised 17% of the community group, 7.6% of the hospital group and only 2.2% of the shared care group (p=0.00005).

Analysis of the care women actually received according to the type of clinic they attended revealed significant differences in all factors with the community clinics seeming the most successful. Differences were most striking with reassurance and emotional support, having one's questions answered and procedures explained, and the opportunity to see a woman doctor. The difference was least marked with privacy which was generally well provided at all the clinics.

Similarly, if one takes into account women's prior expectations, there were significant differences between women receiving the three main types of antenatal care. The differences were most striking with reassurance and emotional support, receiving expert care, seeing the same person each time and being able to see a woman doctor. In each case, those having community based antenatal care were least likely to be disappointed and more likely to be pleasantly surprised by their experiences at the clinic than those having hospital based or shared care.

Obstetric outcome

Analysis of obstetric data by the type of antenatal care received revealed that those women who received their antenatal care in the community showed small but significant differences from the others. They were more likely to have a normal delivery (76.1%) and less likely to have a Caesarean section (10.8%) than those in the hospital (72.8%:18.5%) or shared care groups (71.7%:17.8%). They were less likely to have a preterm birth (community vs hospital vs shared = 3.5%: 9.3%: 4.2%: p=0.03) and less likely to have a baby weighing under 2500g (4.9%: 11.9%: 6.6%: p=0.03). There were no significant differences between the groups in terms of labour onset (spontaneous onset of labour rate in community vs hospital vs shared = 72%: 65%: 68%: p=0.1), length of labour (labour of 8 hours or less = 67%: 73%: 70%: p=0.2), analgesia used (no analgesia or Entonox alone = 60%: 46%: 51%: p=0.1), 5 minute Apgar score[5] (score of 9-10 = 92%: 93%: 94%: p=0.6), birthweight centile (less than 10th centile = 7%: 12%: 9%: p=0.5) or subsequent infant feeding (breast feeding rates = 44%: 35%: 41%: p=0.2). Important explanatory variables such as smoking and body-mass index did not differ between the groups. It is also important to remember that women receiving hospital based care were not at higher risk than the others but were in that group simply because their GP did not offer an antenatal service.

---

5   *The Apgar score gives a new born baby a number according to its physical condition, taking into account its heart rate, respiratory effort, muscle tone, reflex irritability and skin colour. A healthy baby's Apgar score at 5 minutes of age will be 8-10. Scores of less than 7 mean that the baby needs resuscitation and close observation and may be predictive of future developmental delay.*

Women's preferences

When women were asked where they would prefer to go for antenatal care, over half preferred their GP's surgery, not only because of convenience but for the chance of personal care by familiar people. 20% chose a hospital clinic and 6% chose a community midwives' clinic. 4% chose shared care, a surprisingly low figure considering this is the most common form of antenatal care in the borough. A similar query concerning preferred staff had even more striking results. In answer to the question `If you could choose just one person to look after you throughout your pregnancy, who would it be?' 55% chose a midwife and 20% chose their GP. 10% chose a hospital doctor and 5% chose a consultant. It should be made clear that those who chose a hospital doctor did so because of one person they had met with whom they had established a rapport. Hospital doctors were not necessarily chosen for their expertise but because they seemed to be people whom some women at least felt they could trust.

Discussion

Women in East London have high expectations of the antenatal services. Some would assert that they expect too much, but since the specific factors examined in the study form what most would call acceptable care, it is a pity that women are being disappointed. The majority of pregnant women require understanding, patience and minimal intervention during their pregnancies. To quote Professor Chamberlain (1991):

> *'there are two classes of women: the larger requiring support but not much intervention and the other needing the full range of diagnostic and therapeutic measures as in any other branch of medicine. To distinguish between the two is the aim of well run antenatal care'.*

by Ruth Cochrane

The most striking shortfall between expectation and experience related to seeing the same person at each visit and receiving information on baby care. It could be argued that the latter issue is covered at parentcraft classes. In Tower Hamlets, these are attended by only 38% of women and are not routinely offered to those who already have children. However, the issue of continuity of carer is one that could be tackled by the clinic given sufficient forethought. This is important for over three-quarters of the women questioned and yet is a feature of the clinic for less than 10% of them, the majority of whom attend a community based clinic.

The benefits of community antenatal clinics in terms of women's satisfaction have not been won at the expense of good obstetric care. Rather than simple 'doing no harm' (Taylor, 1982) the reverse is the case, but to flourish such schemes require a change in the emphasis of maternity care from the hospital to the community.

Women perceive GPs and midwives as possessing listening ears and seek to use their understanding and empathy to alleviate small, apparently inconsequential worries as well as answering questions directly related to pregnancy. Midwives in particular are seen as important in this context: one woman in the study said:

'I don't like to bother them at the hospital with my little worries as they're always so busy but I feel I can talk to the midwife'.

The belief that the midwife is the appropriate person to care for normal pregnancy and labour is widely held in Tower Hamlets. One woman in answer to the question about choice of carer said:

'Of course I'd have a midwife — a doctor couldn't deliver it could he?'

This preference could have profound implications for the way in which antenatal care is arranged in the future. More midwife clinics could be offered and those GPs who undertake antenatal care should be given more support and encouragement. To achieve these two objectives would require changes in recruitment and training.

What is interesting about the survey results is that the local midwives' self-perceived low status is at odds with the esteem in which they are held by local women. One could thus predict that any change to enhance the role of the midwife in antenatal care, aiming to render the service more relevant, efficient and user-friendly would meet with local approval. There would be wider implications for obstetricians, as with enough women transferred from the hospital to the midwives' clinic, doctors could concentrate on those women needing specialist advice.

Antenatal care has been with us for 75 years but we are still making mistakes. Hospital specialists have adopted new technologies and marginalised the GP and community midwife. If women are to receive the care they need, expect and want, our undergraduate and postgraduate training schedules should take more account of women's priorities and less of poorly scrutinised, unscientific obstetric rituals.

Having said that there is a potential conflict between offering women a choice in antenatal care and performing a properly controlled trial of different forms of care. In some ways the benefits of local, convenient, personalised care are so self-apparent that a formal study would be unnecessary. The importance of this research is to demonstrate that these forms of antenatal care incur no obstetric risk.

The main problems encountered in this study were the logistical difficulties of addressing a large number of women in a multi-ethnic area using face-to-face interviews with a single researcher. This method was chosen to reduce interview bias and to encourage women to discuss their ideas and experiences honestly. It was also felt to be important that the interviewer was not identified as a carer within the service but instead was an objective researcher. An alternative format would be to conduct a postal survey as described by Cartwright (1987). Whilst not suitable for Tower Hamlets, such a study would be workable in more literate areas.

Qualitative rather than quantitative research would have

necessitated recording interviews for later transcription and may also have posed difficulties for subsequent computer analysis. Our intention was to include a large number of women rather than to receive detailed information from a smaller sample.

Conclusion

This study involved a large number of women and only one researcher for the majority of the time. Given the study's financial constraints, a smaller sample would have made the process less unwieldy. If carried out in a different area, preliminary allocation of women to one of the three types of antenatal care in a random way would be a more scientific approach.

Women in Tower Hamlets have a wide choice of types of antenatal care. They have high but understandable expectations of the antenatal services. The service fails them in several ways but overall that failure is least apparent within a community based scheme. The main implication of the study is therefore that community based antenatal care should be enhanced where appropriate as it is acceptable to women and does not confer any obstetric risk. Ideally, antenatal care for the majority of women should involve visits to their GP's surgery to see a midwife who has access to obstetric help as and when necessary. This demonstrates the study's other main implication for service provision, that community based care can help prevent the deskilling of midwives and allow them more professional autonomy. Consumer-orientated research is vital to ensure that a satisfactory service is provided, and the innumerable rituals of maternity care should be subjected to randomised control trials (Enkin *et al*, 1989). We should listen to those for whom the service was established and respect them as individuals, recalling the following words (Browne, 1935) from almost 60 years ago:

> 'in the antenatal clinic, there should be no such thing as mass production'.

References

Bracken MB (1989) Reporting observational studies. *Brit J Obs Gyn* **96**: 383-88

Browne FJ (1935) *Antenatal and postnatal care*. Churchill, London

Carey S, Shukur A (1985) A profile of the Bangladeshi community in East London. *New Community* **12** (3): 405-17

Cartwright A (1987) Monitoring maternity services by postal questionnaires to mothers. *Health Trends* **19**: 19-20

Chamberlain G (1991) Organisation of antenatal care. *Brit Med J* **302**: 647-50

Comaroff J (1977) Conflicting paradigms of pregnancy; managing ambiguity in neonatal encounters. In: Davis A, Horobin G (eds) *Medical Encounters*. Croom Helm, London

Dixon WJ (1990). *BMDP Statistical Software Manual*. University of California Press, Berkeley CA

Enkin M, Keirse MJNC, Chalmers I (1989) *Effective care in pregnancy and childbirth*. Oxford University Press, Oxford

Garcia J (1982) Women's views of antenatal care. In: Enkin M and Chalmers I (eds), *Effectiveness and satisfaction in antenatal care*, Spastics International Medical Publications: Heinemann, London

McKee I (1984) Community antenatal care: the Sighthill community antenatal care scheme. In: Zander L and Chamberlain G (eds), *Pregnancy care for the 1980s, Royal Society of Medicine and Macmillan Press, London*

Microwriter Systems PLC (1988 *Agenda User's Guide*, 2 Wandle Way, Willow Lane, Mitcham, Surrey

Norusis MJ (1986) *SPSS-PC+ for the IBM PC. SPSS Inc, 444 North Michigan Avenue, Chicago, Illinois*

Oakley A (1979). *Becoming a mothe. Martin Robinson, Oxford*

Porter M, MacIntyre S (1984) What is, must be best: a research note on conservative or deferential responses to antenatal care provision. *Soc Sci Med* **19**: 1197-200

Reid ME, Gutteridge S, McIlwaine G M (1983) *A comparison of the delivery of antenatal care between a hospital and a peripheral clinic.* Health Services Research Committee, Scottish Home and Health Department

Reid ME, McIlwaine GM (1980) Consumer opinion of a hospital antenatal clinic. *Soc Sci Med*, **14a**, 363–68

Taylor A (1986) Maternity services: the consumer's view. *J Roy Coll Gen Pract* **36**: 157–60

Taylor RW (1984) Community based specialist antenatal care services. In: Zander L, Chamberlain G (eds), *Pregnancy care for the 1980s.* Royal Society of Medicine and Macmillan Press, London

Widgery D (1991) *Some lives! A GP's East End.* Sinclair-Stevenson, London

William S, Dickson D, Forbes J *et al* (1989) An evaluation of community antenatal care. *Midwifery* **5**: 63–8

Zander LI, Watson M, Taylor RW, Morrell DC (1978) Integration of general practitioner and specialist antenatal care. *J Roy Coll Gen Pract* **28**: 455–58

CHAPTER SEVEN:
SERVICES for PEOPLE who have been SEXUALLY ABUSED

*Sharon Gray, Marietta Higgs
and Keith Pringle*

Abstract

This chapter describes two comparative surveys of services for people who have experienced sexual abuse: one aimed at statutory agencies, the other at adult survivors of such abuse. The research method used for both surveys was the self-completed questionnaire. The reasons for the choice of this particular method are discussed. The capacity of such a method to produce qualitative as well as quantitative data is considered as well as its ability to contribute to research which has an overtly anti-oppressive purpose

In terms of results, tentative conclusions are suggested and many controversial issues for debate as well as for further research are highlighted

Why we chose to research this issue?

Child Abuse Listening Line (CALL)[1] is a voluntary organisation, based in Northumberland, which seeks to fill gaps in provision for adults who have experienced sexual abuse. In 1991 CALL felt this

1   *Anyone wishing to contact CALL should write to Judith Oliver, Chairperson, CALL, 96 Sweethope Avenue, Ashington, Northumberland, NE63 9PW*

task would be assisted by researching into the services which are available to survivors and identifying those which should be developed. The basic idea (formulated by Sharon Gray, at that time Director of CALL) was that an audit of services provided by major agencies for children and for adults who have been sexually abused should be carried out. Moreover, she suggested that this should be paralleled by a survey of adult survivors' views on resources which were available as well as those which they felt were desirable. In making this suggestion Sharon was aware that in the vast majority of cases the abuse experienced by the survivors would typically have occurred in childhood and/or adolescence (see Glaser and Frosh, 1993; for an excellent general summary of data on the characteristics of sexual abuse). Thus a survey of adult survivors' views on services could also cast light on what agencies told us about their resources for children as well as those for adults.

The research team

It was decided that two of CALL's practice consultants and Sharon would undertake this research. The personalities, philosophies, and backgrounds of researchers can have a major bearing on the way research is shaped and executed. Consequently, we will summarise some relevant details about the three researchers who are also the authors of this chapter.

We brought different experiences and, to some extent, perspectives to the task. Sharon, who is a survivor, works as a therapist, primarily with adult survivors using a child advocacy model (drawing very much on the work of Alice Miller), and as a trainer for various statutory and voluntary organisations — she is also active in various community/voluntary groups. Marietta is a paediatrician who also works with several community groups/organisations in the North East of England which promote awareness about the issue of sexual abuse and the need for professionals and non-professionals to act together to assist survivors. Keith teaches and researches applied social studies in a local university, having practised as a qualified social worker for ten years — he also works with a variety of voluntary groups seeking to break down the barriers of professional/non-professional in service provision and his predominant approach to the issue of sexual abuse is a pro-feminist one.

The three researchers had known each other for a considerable time and were clear about their respective and differing value bases: for instance, we were (and still are) aware of our divergent views about the importance of the feminist perspective in relation to sexual abuse. We also knew we were united by a person-centred approach to sexual abuse services and by a desire to co-ordinate provision available from non-professionals and professionals.

Inevitably our philosophies and interests influenced the shape of the research process. This was so where our perspectives coincided: for instance, the whole project was deliberately survivor-focused. However, the differences between us also had an impact. One example was the way we chose which questions to pursue, given that the number of issues we could have explored was legion. It is fair to say that Keith was particularly keen to investigate factors related to gender and 'race' and some compromise had to be struck between his interests and those of Sharon and Marietta.

It should be noted that all three of us are white. This imbalance in terms of ethnic origin is unfortunately common in the area of sexual abuse research and has certainly skewed the current literature on the subject (see the discussion in Wilson, 1993). We did have some awareness of black issues in this field and incorporated elements of that awareness into the research format. Nevertheless, it is true to say that a black perspective on the topics raised in the research was not as prominent as perhaps it should have been.

Initial discussions among the three of us were based on Sharon's original idea of administering by post self-completion questionnaires about services provided and required to both adult survivors and to agencies. This would allow us to compare and contrast the responses. We already had an hypothesis (based on our own experiences) that the services provided by large agencies often did not match, in scale or quality, the needs of service users. Although we tried not to prejudge the outcome and maintained a keen awareness of how the form of our questions had the potential to shape the results, we were very clear about what we were testing and what we thought **might** transpire.

Choice of research methods

From the outset the form of the research was partly dictated by an awareness of the possibility that the results could be used to lobby large agencies and central government for a change in the pattern of service provision — if the need for such a change was confirmed by the results. Previous experience of dealing with large, local agencies led us to believe that research with a quantitative or quasi-quantitative format was more likely to be given credibility by them than research using purely qualitative methods (for instance, in-depth interviews/discussions with a small number of survivors). Their privileging of quantitative methods seems to originate in a desire for 'hard facts', although (as we make clear below) we ourselves would regard such a connection as being simplistic. Nevertheless, given our purpose, their privileging of quantitative research did partly influence our decision to conduct a 'trawl' of a relatively large number of informants using self-completion questionnaires sent to them.

A self-completion questionnaire survey also seemed an appropriate research strategy on other counts. For instance, the resources available to us were very limited. The research was funded on a 'shoe-string', CALL paying for stationary costs etc. and the researchers working in their own time for no payment. Although no attempt was made to seek wider funding in this case, some of us had previous experience of the difficulty in obtaining independent resources for research on sexual abuse where that research is located outside the large agencies and within a non-professional or unconventional framework.

In a sense, the problem about obtaining funding is symptomatic of a wider difficulty in gaining recognition within the field of sexual abuse for non-professional service provision and for research which may challenge the Establishment within child welfare services. It is a tribute to non-professionals, survivors, and self-help groups that they manage to achieve so much, frequently in the face of hostility from professionals and indifference from resource gate-keepers. The reasons for this polarisation are deep and varied: the subject still awaits proper study. Pringle, 1990, 1993; Armstrong, 1991; Hudson, 1992 and Wilson, 1993; provide initial exploration of the issue. A vital factor seems to be the intrinsic importance of political issues to the field of sexual abuse and the challenge which the subject therefore presents to power hierarchies in society, including those of gender and class (see Kidd and Pringle, 1988; for a more extended discussion of this political dimension).

Returning to our discussion about the rationale for using self-completion questionnaires, that decision needs to be set in context. We did value for its own sake the information that a survey might throw up about the services available to survivors. But it would be disingenuous to pretend that we were uninfluenced in our choice of research method by factors such as cost and 'political credibility' — factors which some positivists might regard as methodologically impure (see Fay, 1975; and the discussion in May, 1993).

In recent years the positivist concept of value-free research, particularly in the social sciences, has been seriously qualified — partly due to the insights offered by feminist writers (see for example Roberts, 1981; Stanley and Wise, 1983; Everitt *et al*, 1992 and May, 1993). One feminist response to the inescapability of 'bias' in research is to be as aware (and as open) as possible about the agendas operating in each research process: which is our preference, too, and we are seeking to achieve it here.

In the light of what we have just said, it may be thought ironic that we chose a research method (i.e. the self-completion questionnaire) which has in the past been so closely associated with 'objective' and positivist research.

It is also ironic because all three of us (in differing ways) have a clear commitment to the value of hearing the direct voice of the survivor of sexual abuse. In our view it is impossible to over-rate the power of the truth when a survivor speaks out about her/his own experiences. That power, rather than the effort of professionals, has been the real engine for meaningful change in the way our society reacts to sexual abuse (see Armstrong, 1991) — though professionals may still have an important enabling role to play (Pringle, 1993).

This commitment to the voice of the survivor is closely related to the 'standpoint epistemology' to be found in some feminist models of research (Roberts, 1981) which generally sets great store on the value of qualitative evidence. All three of us share that respect for qualitative methodology — and recognise that, generally speaking, the voice of the survivor is best heard in research terms via semi-structured interviewing or by using focus groups.

Once again, therefore, it might be argued that our use of a self-completion questionnaire format for reasons of cost and political expediency was a hostage to positivist research methodologies: and that thereby we have contradicted our commitment to the voice of the survivor and betrayed the anti-oppressive perspective which we hold on the issue of sexual abuse (La Fontaine, 1990; Glaser and Frosh, 1993).

We would maintain that this is an over-simplistic analysis for several reasons. First of all, we do not believe positivism and quantitative analysis are always synonymous. Moreover, the alleged dichotomy between qualitative and quantitative methods can also be misleading: it is possible to combine the two. Everitt *et al* (1992) explore both these issues further. We hope the account in this chapter will provide a practical demonstration how a method such as a self-completion questionnaire can incorporate qualitative as well as quantitative elements — and be used with some, albeit limited, success in the context of an anti-oppressive project.

Designing and administering the questionnaires

Having decided upon the research method which we would use, we then had to consider the scope of the project. Once again, resource constraints affected the size of the exercise. Our first intention had been to conduct a national survey: we soon realised our focus would have to be narrowed to match the limited time and money available to us. We decided instead to concentrate on services within the North of England (from Cleveland to the Scottish border and from the North Sea to Cumbria).

When we started to think about the nature of the questionnaires which we would devise, we quickly recognised the one for adult survivors would need to be rather different in design from that for agencies and it may be useful to consider the reasons behind our decision.

First and most important, we recognised that although the form of information required from both sets of respondents was similar (i.e. What services are available? What should be available?), the nature of that information would be very different. On the one hand, it was not unreasonable to expect much of the agency data to be relatively hard and factual (if you accept those terms). On the other hand, the survivors' responses might well be valuable not only for their factual content but also for their personal perspective (e.g. How did it feel to be a consumer of particular services?). Consequently, we wanted to provide a somewhat less structured questionnaire format for the survivors with more opportunity for open-ended remarks about their views. The agency questionnaire needed to be more structured to elicit both a full range of information and to ensure consistency in the areas covered by each agency so that comparisons between their responses might be made easier and more valid.

This dichotomy in questionnaire design was reinforced by our perception of the different levels of motivation which might exist between agency and survivor respondents. We felt it was reasonable to assume many survivor respondents would be impelled by a very personal and powerful commitment to answer the questionnaire i.e. that their motivation would often be high. In that context, we assumed they would persevere with a relatively open-ended questionnaire which might take considerable time to fill in and would entail a fair degree of involvement.

By contrast, we assumed that many welfare professionals responding to their questionnaire might, quite realistically, regard it as a relatively low priority in relation to the pressure of immediate tasks which they also faced. This provided another reason for designing a more structured questionnaire for agencies which was quicker to complete and required perhaps less analysis by respondents than would be the case for the survivors' questionnaire.

Detailed structure of questionnaires.

(a) Adult survivors' questionnaire (see Appendix 1)

Information was sought about the nature of the abuse experienced by the adult survivor because it was felt potential links between this data and the types of assistance preferred by survivors might be illuminating. For instance, was there any link between the gender of the abuser and the gender of therapist preferred by a survivor?

Survivors' views on the efficacy of the help they received was obviously also vital — particularly where different sources of help had been used over time and it was possible for survivors to make a comparison. We suggested variables which survivors might consider and these were drawn from our own experience of working with survivors. Some of the variables related to factors such as: the differential impact of statutory/non-statutory provision; assistance provided by other survivors (whether 'professionals' or not) compared to the value of assistance from non-survivors. In addition, however, we regarded it as vital to provide, within the structure, ample opportunity for each survivor to define the variables which **they** felt to be important and to comment on them.

The final area of the questionnaire focused on survivors' views regarding what ought to be available to them as opposed to that which actually existed. Again the questionnaire consisted of a combination of suggested topics for comment and an invitation to survivors to construct their own topics and priorities with space for open-ended responses.

(b) Agency questionnaire (see Appendix 2)

This started with a written preamble by one of us (KP) explaining the precise purposes of the survey, acknowledging the time pressures on those to whom the questionnaire was being sent, and emphasising how the information garnered might be useful to agency respondents and survivors. Instructions were given on how to complete the questionnaire, stressing the ease of the task. This preamble was designed to increase the likelihood of agency recipients responding, given the other demands on their time noted above. Unfortunately, due again to lack of resources, it was not feasible to enclose a pre-paid return envelope with questionnaires.

There were four parts to this questionnaire: in three of them the same questions were asked in relation to three different scenarios i.e. services available in cases of (i) child sexual abuse (ii) adults sexually abused in childhood (iii) adults sexually abused in adulthood. The fourth part was a generic section seeking information about gaps in provision, future training needs, and underlying philosophies of provision.

The first three sections elicited responses about issues such as: the kinds of assistance provided to survivors (i.e. individual, family, groupwork); the ages of survivors catered for; whether assistance was provided to others involved such as family / friends of survivors, abusers, family / friends of abusers; services provided to black people; the professional label of those providing services (e.g. 'social worker', 'psychiatrist', 'psychologist' etc.). Many of these issues were explored via tick lists or requests for one-word answers. That latter strategy sometimes precluded gaining the depth of response which we might have liked — but, as noted above, it had the advantage of being quick to fill in which seemed to us to be an important consideration for many professionals.

The final, fourth, section of the agency questionnaire was shorter but also more open-ended, partly because we did not feel the information required here could be dealt with by tick lists.

The method of distribution of both questionnaires requires some comment. As regards the survivors' questionnaires, CALL sent these out to the adult survivors known to it and to other survivor and self-help groups, there being considerable contact and, indeed, overlap of membership between these groups. Clearly, such a method of distribution could to some extent bias the results. For instance, survivors using survivors' groups might tend to be those whose needs had not previously been met by statutory agencies. This, then, might produce an over-negative picture of statutory provision. On the other hand, it could be argued that such people are precisely those whose views are most relevant in order to make statutory provision as comprehensive as possible.

The distribution of agency questionnaires was more systematic, using directories to target relevant offices in the region. Originally, the target group was intended to be very wide: social services team offices and specialist staff; relevant points in the health service; probation services; education; large voluntary organisations. However, due to resource problems we had to narrow the field and a good coverage was only achieved in terms of social services and health.

Results

Given the space available here and the fact that the focus of this publication is on research methods, we will only provide a summary of the results and their implications. For a fuller discussion of these issues see the report to the originating organisation, CALL (Gray *et al*. forthcoming).

(a) Agency responses

Overall 29 of these were returned. This represented a reasonable spread across social services departments in the region . Admittedly only thirteen were returned out of thirty one sent out; but of those thirteen, most were responses from child protection co-ordinators for the local authorities who were able to give an overall picture of the services for the whole of the area for which they were responsible. As a result, we have quite an accurate picture of the services provided by local authorities across the North East region. The outcome for the health service was eight responses out of forty one sent, which is clearly less satisfactory but still enables a degree of comment to be made. The remainder of returns were from services such as education and probation where the distribution of questionnaires had been admittedly patchy. Obviously the number of returns limits how far the results can be generalised: however for social services, and to a lesser extent health, the results would seem to have some validity. The better return rate of social services may in part be due to the fact that, as noted already, the agency questionnaire was issued with a preamble by the researcher with a social work background (KP) who is relatively familiar to the agencies in that sector.

A second limiting factor which needs to be acknowledged is that of time. The data presented was collected mainly in 1992 and the first half of 1993. As always, a time-lag exists between collection, analysis, and then publication. This process was exacerbated by the fact that the research was carried out largely in the researchers' own time. In an area as fast-moving as that of sexual abuse, such a time gap might distort the current situation. Having said that, our personal experience suggests that the picture painted by the results is not markedly different from the present one in the North East of England.

There is a final, rather obvious, issue which could distort results: perhaps some respondents were not giving completely honest responses. For example, some statutory authorities might be very wary of admitting gaps in provision, particularly in such a highly charged area of work as sexual abuse. There is no doubt that certain responses portrayed a picture which is far more positive than we know, from our own experience as practitioners, to actually be the case in some localities.

This highlights a weakness of the research. Since self-completion questionnaires will often have a propensity for such corruption by respondents, it is useful to build in a second line of enquiry as a check on results — perhaps the opportunity for in-depth discussions with a cross-section of respondents. We neither had the finances nor the time to provide this back-up. Of course that checking strategy would not have been fool-proof even if we could have afforded it.

Moreover, by contrast we should also add that some agency respondents seemed to be remarkably honest about their situation. For instance take these two comments, both from major providers of services:

> "*The scale of need for children and adults who have been abused is far greater than the provision of services for them.*"

> There is a "*...dismal lack of services for adolescents who have been abused.*"

Bearing in mind these three provisos about the validity of our agency data, we now summarise significant results in each section of the agency questionnaire. We will discuss some of the implications as we proceed.

(1)   Services for children sexually abused.

Statutory agencies seemed to concentrate on investigation and assessment of `cases`, rather than on longer-term, therapeutic, assistance. This was not an unexpected finding, given that non-statutory providers such as Rape Crisis Centres have long reported a massive demand for therapeutic help which far outstrips their resources. Indeed, it was partly to fill this very gap that several small-scale independent, survivor-focused services had developed in the North East of England during the late 1980's, such as CALL, Childcentre, Cleveland Against Child Abuse, Wear Women In Need (now a major provider), and Justice for Abused Children.

They also developed because the large voluntary child-care organisations in the region similarly provided only limited therapeutic services of a focused nature in the field of sexual abuse: about four such projects are run by various organisations — and these tend to be part-funded by local authority or health service resources.

Facilities in the statutory agencies for abusers who are children also seemed very limited according to our questionnaires, though this result might have been distorted by lack of data from probation services.

By contrast, our results do suggest considerable provision for non-abusing parents. Unfortunately, the questionnaire did not ask whether such provision was separate from the service to the child. Research is increasingly making it clear that support to non-abusing parents is absolutely crucial to the future well-being of the child and that it is best provided separately. In other words, you may need two professionals for each situation (a support worker for the parent and a key-worker for the child survivor) rather than one. To agencies this may often seem costly in the short-run: it is however essential (see Hooper, 1993). The lack of exploration of that issue in the agency questionnaire may distort our findings. More distortion could also have been introduced by some agencies' reluctance to be sufficiently open about the true situation: once again our own practice experience across the region is that support for non-abusing parents is less impressive than the account given in some of the questionnaires would lead us to believe.

Agency services for the family of the abuser, whether child or adult, are virtually non-existent apart from provision by one small voluntary organisation which has some statutory support.

There was a surprising lack of groupwork support in agencies for child and adolescent survivors compared to individual and family work. The reasons for this could be several. First of all, if most statutory work is centred on investigation and assessment rather than on longer-term assistance, such a finding might well be anticipated as groupwork tends to be primarily a therapeutic activity.

There may, however, be a more interesting explanation as well. Later in the questionnaire we asked respondents if their work had any particular theoretical underpinning. Only one respondent mentioned a feminist approach. Although provision of groupwork is not confined to services influenced by a feminist perspective (see Bentovim *et al*, 1988), nevertheless that perspective is particularly conducive to groupwork methods given its' potential for empowerment (see Butler and Wintram, 1991). So lack of groupwork may partly reflect the relatively small influence of a feminist approach on services in this region. Such a picture is not characteristic of all other regions in Britain: in some areas of the country a feminist perspective is more influential in the provision of services (see Feminist Review, 1988; for an example).

Turning to the important issue of preventive work, agencies made no secret of their lack of provision, although it partly depended on how they defined 'prevention': some authorities saw the avoidance of further sexual abuse as preventive. Even so, no matter how it was defined, the picture regarding prevention in the responses was bleak.

Equally bleak was the almost total lack of provision for black children who are abused, despite considerable evidence in the literature of the desperate need for such services (see Ahmad, 1990;

Pringle, 1993 and Wilson, 1993). The most chilling aspect of the results was that the majority of agency respondents did not even bother to answer the question relating to this issue in the survey. That remarkable negligence was also replicated in the later sections of the questionnaire dealing with services for adults abused in childhood and those abused in adulthood. One conclusion may be that this most visible of minorities in our society is apparently invisible when it comes to making resources available to them. A change in policy by statutory agencies to meet the needs of black people may be urgently required. A first step would be for agencies to ask the black communities what form of services would be most useful to them.

(2) Services for adults abused in childhood

More or less the same results occurred as in (1) above — except that services were much smaller across the board for this user group. Partners of abused adults received particularly little support.

(3) Services for adults abused in adulthood

Statutory provision for these users was extremely limited indeed. A significant point was made by one agency respondent who noted that services for such people were only likely to be freed up if they themselves had children who might be deemed 'at risk'. Once again, non-abusing partners of abused adults were scarcely catered for.

As noted above, a general enquiry was made at the end of the questionnaire about theoretical frameworks used by agencies in their provision of services. What emerged from the results was a remarkable lack of such frameworks within statutory services. The overall picture was of relatively *'ad hoc'* service provision with few theoretical principles. The most common frameworks in use cited by respondents were 'eclectic' (without further explanation of that term) or 'Children Act/child protection procedures'. The latter response is particularly worrying given that neither the Act nor protection procedures provide specific guidance about how to engage survivors in longer-term therapeutic work. Moreover, the Children Act is itself riven by theoretical and practical contradictions: Frost (1992) and Allen (1992) begin to provide a much-needed critique of the Act. The conclusion to be drawn from the agency responses is that we may need to question the coherence of many of those therapeutic services which statutory agencies do manage to provide. Further debate and research on this subject is clearly warranted.

Agency respondents were finally asked to suggest areas of work which required further development or for which they would like more training. The results were varied but interesting. The most common area identified by agencies as requiring urgent development was work with sexual abusers (particularly adolescents) to attempt to limit their potential for re-offending. Other suggestions for development of services included: worker support; adult survivors found in adult services (for instance those survivors with difficulties in the area of mental health, or who were older people, or people with learning disabilities); training for managers; training in the provision of therapeutic assistance to survivors. Many of these seem useful ideas and reflect wider research studies: Glaser and Frosh (1993) and Finkelhor (1986) provide a summary of those findings.

The emphasis on work with sexual abusers requires some comment. No one would deny the need for this activity if it results in fewer people being abused in the future. The efficacy of work with abusers is, however, still open to debate. Moreover, the concentration of statutory agencies on developing work with abusers raises an issue about the balance of scarce resources channelled to different sectors within the field of sexual abuse: how much should be devoted to the direct needs of survivors and how much to abusers? This is a particularly pertinent question to ask when one examines the results of the questionnaires completed by survivors.

(b) Survivors responses

There were 36 of these received back out of a total of 52 sent out. Once again it would not be appropriate to regard this sample size as allowing definitive judgements about services provided. Nevertheless, these responses do enable us to make some tentative suggestions which need to be debated and followed up by larger-scale surveys.

Of the respondents, only six were male. We know from prevalence surveys (e.g. Finkelhor *et al*, 1990; and Kelly *et al*, 1991) that the number of males sexually abused is far higher than our data would suggest, though still less than the number of females abused. It may well be that the absence of males in our survey partly reflects the well-known greater reluctance of men and boys to disclose their abuse (see La Fontaine, 1990; especially pp85–88). It might also be a function of the lack of independent survivor-focused services for men.

The questionnaire did ask whether survivors were black or white. Only two respondents were black: one defined herself as being of dual heritage, the other as Asian (Sikh). Again, this is a result which must cause concern. As we noted above, agencies made virtually no provision for black survivors. Now we see that black people do not appear to turn to established survivor-focused and self-help groups for assistance either.

A major issue for further research follows from these findings on black survivors: why do many statutory and survivor-focused services seem not to cater for black people? Is it because those services discriminate? Is it because the provision of the services is largely in the hands of white people and that in itself is off-putting to some potential black service users? Or is it perhaps because research by us as white people may have omitted inadvertently any services for black people which do exist? Based on the small amount of material available on this topic, our suspicion is that all these factors probably play some part (see Wilson, 1993; for an excellent discussion of the subject, particularly pp8-9 and 167-74). As was noted earlier, it is vital that services are provided which will meet the needs of the black communities and the views of the latter on the form of those services should be sought as a first step in that process.

The gender of abusers was also a significant factor in this survey for several reasons. Of the female survivors, the vast majority were abused by males: four reported abuse perpetrated by a male and female jointly; none reported abuse by a lone female. Of the six male respondents, two reported abuse by a man and woman jointly, three were abused by a male alone, and one by a female alone. Such gender proportions are more or less in line with the results of large prevalence surveys reported in the literature (Finkelhor *et al*, 1990; and Kelly, 1991) except that in those more reliable surveys the number of males abused by a lone male is even higher.

For the purposes of our survey the information we had about gender of perpetrators was particularly important in terms of the kind of therapist with whom survivors said they would prefer to work. The vast majority of our respondents said they would want a female therapist, with a few indicating they had no preference. These findings held true for male and female respondents: of the six male survivors, two expressed no preference about gender either way, and four actually said they would prefer a female therapist. Only one respondent out of the thirty six said they would prefer a male therapist: a female survivor who had in fact been abused by a male perpetrator. Although we have to be careful about over-generalising given the relatively small size of our sample, these results clearly require further debate and research in terms of what they may tell us about the potential role (or possibly lack of role) for males as therapists (see Pringle, 1992 and Frosh, 1988; for further discussion of this highly controversial issue).

Many respondents had experience of both statutory and survivor-focused voluntary services. The vast majority expressed a strong preference for non-statutory provision. Only nine respondents said statutory services would be acceptable to them and eight of those made that judgement in terms of expressing no preference between either statutory or voluntary provision. The design of the questionnaire did not allow direct exploration of the reasons for this finding, which in retrospect is unfortunate. However, some of the reasons can be surmised from other responses made by survivors in their questionnaires.

For instance, another striking result was the preference expressed by the vast majority of respondents for therapists who were themselves survivors of sexual abuse. In self-help groups and small survivor-focused independent charities, therapists are often open about the abusive experiences they may have themselves endured in their own lives. Within the statutory services those workers and therapists who may themselves be survivors of sexual abuse do not normally divulge this for a variety of reasons: partly because it is often regarded by agencies as being 'unprofessional' to do so; and also because such survivors often fear that they would be regarded as less suitable for the work they do by their colleagues and managers (see Pringle, 1993 and Wilson, 1993; for further discussion). It is important to stress that there is no evidence that survivors are less effective as professionals in working with sexual abuse: indeed, in our experience many of the most gifted professionals in this field are actually survivors themselves.

This difference towards self-disclosure may be one reason why survivors in our research expressed such a strong preference for non-statutory services. Significantly, that minority of respondents who did say they would accept professional help were virtually unanimous in stipulating that the professional had also to be a survivor of sexual abuse. In terms of building alliances between professional and non-professional sources of assistance for survivors, professionals who are also survivors may have a crucial role to play (Pringle, 1993) and their situation therefore warrants further debate and research.

The major reason why so many survivors preferred non-statutory provision may be connected with the form of assistance offered to respondents. Over half the survivors said they wanted open access to therapists and almost all indicated that therapeutic help should be available as long as the individual survivor felt she/he needed it. This implies the survivor should have considerable, possibly total, control over the shape of the assistance they receive. Such conditions are increasingly unlikely within provision made available by social services departments or even the health service due to resource pressures and the increasingly bureaucratic form in which such provision is framed. By contrast, small survivor-focused and self-help services do tend to place the survivor in considerable control over the therapeutic process and offer more flexibility in terms of provision.

A further mis-match between statutory agency services and those preferred by survivors in our two questionnaires centres on the types of provision available. We noted above that agencies tended to provide services less in the form of groupwork and much more in the shape of individual and family work. In one important respect preferences stated by survivors were diametrically opposed to that balance of provision. Whilst twenty two survivors did want individual assistance, only six wanted help delivered in the form of a family-wide service. By contrast, twenty three respondents expressed a preference for groupwork provision.

This divergence may be partly explained by the nature of our research method. The survivors in our survey were, of course, all adults when they answered the questionnaire, although the vast majority were actually abused in childhood and adolescence. Consequently, it is possible that as adults they no longer saw value in family work though they might have done so earlier in their lives. It would be worth exploring this possibility by further similar research with children and young people who have been sexually abused.

However, in the absence of such research we need to seriously consider the more likely explanation for the disparity of views we have found between agencies and survivors as to the balance of family work and groupwork in service provision:

statutory agencies are not listening to what survivors are telling them and have their own reasons (outlined earlier in this chapter) for putting such emphasis on family work rather than groupwork.

The same mis-match occurs in terms of who receives help. To give one example, over half of our survivors felt their partners needed assistance with their feelings and yet, as we discussed above, agencies made little provision in this respect. Moreover, we could discuss several other similar points of divergence if space allowed (see Gray, Higgs and Pringle [forthcoming] for further details).

The overall impression is that what statutory agencies provide and what adult survivors want are often not the same. It is hardly surprising, then, that survivors look elsewhere to have their needs met.

Implications of this research

As we have said, the small sample size of both sets of our respondents, agencies and survivors, limits the extent to which we can make definitive statements. Nevertheless, there are two major conclusions to be drawn from this research which require further, more large-scale enquiry:

1. There seem to be many major gaps in the provision of statutory agencies. Some of these gaps are perceived by such agencies, others are not.

2. In several important respects, the nature of services provided by agencies appears not to be that preferred by most survivors.

Apart from indicating the direction of future research, our intention is that these two surveys can be directly used to lobby agencies in our region. Our aim is that statutory agencies should reconsider the shape and size of the services they provide as well as increasing their currently meagre financial support to smaller, survivor-focused charities.

How far such a strategy will be successful remains to be seen.

Near the start of this chapter we discussed the various reasons why we chose to use a relatively quantitative research method such as a written questionnaire. One of the reasons related to the perceived greater readiness of bureaucratic agencies to accept data drawn from quantitative rather than qualitative methods. Obviously our success or failure in lobbying agencies using this research may cast light on whether that perception was accurate.

Earlier in the chapter we also mentioned that the distinction between quantitative and qualitative research methods was not always as clear-cut as might be expected. We hope that our account of these two surveys has illustrated this point. Both surveys involved quantitative and qualitative features, and that was particularly true of the survivors' questionnaire. In this manner we hope we can fulfil the political purposes of our research and retain the authentic voice of the survivor which is, in our experience, always the source of true advances made in the field of sexual abuse.

References

Allen N (1992) *Making Sense Of The Children Act*. Longman, London, passim

Ahmad B (1990) *Black Perspectives in Social Work*. Venture Press, Birmingham: pp23–28

Armstrong L (1991) Surviving The Incest Industry. *Trouble And Strife* 21: 29–33

Bentovim A, Elton A, Hildebrand J, Tranter M, Vizard E (eds.) (1988) *Child Sexual Abuse Within The Family: Assessment and Treatment*. Wright, London, passim

Butler S, Wintram C (1991) *Feminist Groupwork*. Sage, London: 5–24

Everitt A, Hardiker P, Littlewood J, Mullender A (1992). *Applied Research For Better Practice*. Macmillan, London: 19–20, passim

Fay B (1975) *Social Theory and Political Practice*. Allen and Unwin, London: 13

by Sharon Gray, Marietta Higgs and Keith Pringle

Feminist Review (1988) **28** passim

Finkelhor D (1986) *Sourcebook On Child Sexual Abuse.* Sage, Newbury Park, California, passim

Finkelhor D, Hotaling G, Lewis I, Smith C (1990) Sexual Abuse in a National Survey of Adult Men And Women. *Child Abus Neg* **14**: 19–28

Frosh S (1988) No Man's Land?: The Role Of Men Working With Sexually Abused Children. *Br J Guid Couns* **16**: 1–10

Frost N (1992) Implementing The Children Act 1989 In A Hostile Climate. In: Carter P, Jeffs T, Smith MK (eds.) *Changing Social Work and Welfare.* Open University, Buckingham: 1–13

Glaser D, Frosh S (1993). *Child Sexual Abuse.* Macmillan, London, passim.

Gray S, Higgs M, Pringle K (forthcoming) *Services for People Who Have Been Sexually Abused: Agency Provision and Survivor Preferences.* Child Abuse Listening Line, Ashington, Northumberland, passim.

Hooper CA (1992) *Mothers Surviving Child Sexual Abuse.* Routledge, London: 164–74

Hudson A (1992) The Child Sexual Abuse 'Industry' and Gender Relations in Social Work. In: Langan M, Day L (eds.) *Women, Oppression and Social Work.* Routledge, London: 129–48

Kelly L, Regan L, Burton S (1991). *An Exploratory Study of the Prevalence of Sexual Abuse in a Sample of 16–21-year-olds.* Polytechnic of North London: 7

Kidd L, Pringle K (1988) The Politics Of Child Sexual Abuse. *Social Work Today* **20**(3): 14–15

La Fontaine J (1990) *Child Sexual Abuse.* Polity Press, Cambridge: 85–91

May T (1993) *Social Research: Issues, Methods and Process.* Open University, Buckingham: 4, 14–18

Pringle K (1990) *Managing To Survive.* Barnardos, Barkingside: 92–93

Pringle K (1992) Child Sexual Abuse Perpetrated By Welfare Personnel And The Problem Of Men. *Critical Soc Policy* **36** passim

Pringle K (1993) Feminist Perspectives on the Way Forward. In: Helm M, Pringle K, Taylor R (eds.) *Surviving Sexual Abuse.* Barnardos,

Barkingside: 85–91

Roberts H (1981) *Doing Feminist Research.* Routledge And Kegan Paul, London, passim.

Stanley L, Wise S (1983) *Breaking Out: Feminist Consciousness and Feminist Research.* Routledge and Kegan Paul, London, passim.

Wilson M (1993) *Crossing The Boundary: Black Women Survive Incest.* Virago, London: 8–9, 157–77

CHAPTER 8
NEGOTIATION and COMPROMISE in RESEARCHING WOMEN'S VIEWS of the CERVICAL SMEAR TEST

Susan Gregory and Linda McKie

Introduction

In this chapter we are seeking to present a realistic portrait of the development and implications of a research project conducted on an intimate area of health screening for women, namely the cervical smear test1. Thus our focus is upon the development process for the project — the processes of negotiation and compromise — rather than the reporting of research results (Gregory and McKie, 1992) 2. Not only is the cervical smear test an intimate matter for many women but it is also a political one. As women's health issues gain prominence on the political agenda the great potential for the treatment and potential cure of abnormal and malignant cells in the cervix belies the continued pattern of approximately 2,000 deaths per annum from cervical cancer. The fact that the cervical smear

---

1   *This portrait of the project is written by two members of a team of four. One of us was involved from the conception of the project, the other commenced work in 1989. Please note that any errors and omissions in this account are those of the authors of this chapter and cannot be attributed to the full research team.*

2   *The results of the project are reported in Gregory and McKie (1992) and McKie (1993a and 1993b).*

test, conducted on a regular basis, can detect early abnormalities and trigger subsequent treatment has promoted a fierce debate concerning the provision of and participation in a national cervical screening service.

The research team, who conducted the research reported in this chapter, were keen to find out what women's views were of the screening service and whether these views bore any relationship to the perceptions commonly employed by some doctors and health planners. A key aim of the project was to involve health workers in both the development and implications of the research ensuring that the views of women were listened to and acted upon. In this chapter we seek to describe the process of negotiating the parameters and conduct of the project and address a number of issues, namely:

1. The debates between the doctors, pathologists, health planners, on the one hand, and social scientists, local community workers and women, on the other, concerning the nature of the research question and conduct of the research;

2. The problems that arose in researching an intimate area of women's lives employing a combination of survey and discussion group methods, and

3. The process of the dissemination of results to women who participated, health professionals, researchers and the research funding body.

The chapter opens with a brief discussion of cervical cancer, the development of screening services and issues concerning the researching of women's health. In the following sections the origins of the project and the process of the research are explored. The chapter concludes with a personal review of the implications of the research process. Throughout the chapter we have attempted to present a realistic and honest picture of a research process which bridged five years of work from it's inception in 1987 to the final analysis of the data in 1992.

Cervical Cancer and Screening Services

Much concern has been expressed on continuing levels of mortality with approximately 2000 women a year in the UK dying from cervical cancer (Central Statistical Office, 1992, p.135). This trend has continued despite the existence of a national screening programme introduced in 1964 which has been amended as part of the new GP. contract (Day, 1989, Dept. of Health, 1989). Current epidemiological work has identified those at particular risk as working class, and older women (Roberts, 1982; Whitehead, 1987). The viruses linked to cervical cancer are sexually transmitted but current treatment has developed in the diagnosis and treatment of women. Given the symptomless nature of the early stage of cervical cancer it is important that women have tests on a regular basis.

However, a reduction in mortality is not the only rationale for providing a screening programme although this is the ultimate goal. The minimisation of morbidity and the enhancement of the effectiveness of treatment, by early intervention, are further goals. Recent figures for Great Britain indicate the continued trend in mortality which must be contrasted with the increasing number of smear tests taken.

Table 8.1: Cervical cancer: deaths and screening

	thousands and percentages		
Great Britain	1981	1984	1988/9
Deaths %	2.2	2.1	2.1
Smears taken— 000s	3,442	3,911	5,032
Smears as % of women aged 15 and over	15.2	17.0	21.5

Source: Central Statistical Office (1992, p135)

Chomet and Chomet (1989, p.132) note that the number of positive smears detected trebled between 1975 and 1985. Whilst the majority of deaths continue to occur amongst older age groups, particularly amongst those who have never had a test (Chamberlain et al, 1984), the majority of abnormal smears are detected in smears from women under 35 (Chomet and Chomet, op. cit.). Such data suggests that without screening and subsequent treatment, the mortality rate would rise. As Posner (1993) notes,

> *"Screening is a public health measure employed to identify disease, or the potential for disease, in the population, so that some form of intervention can take place to try to prevent its development."*

Cervical screening is a form of secondary prevention — an intervention at an early or presymptomatic stage in order to stop further development of a disease — that now forms part of the GP. contract (Dept. of Health, 1990) and recently published health strategies (Dept. of Health, 1992; Scottish Office, 1992).

In the GP contract a financial incentive is linked to local screening provision. Women aged between 25–64 in England and Wales and 20–60 in Scotland were to be invited for a smear test in the five years preceding April 1993. If GPs achieved an 80% goal of women in the target group having a smear test, full payment was made to the practice for this service. If 50% to 79% coverage was achieved, a third of the payment was made and if less than 50% coverage was achieved then no payment was made.

To this incentive scheme must now be added the additional dimension of health care strategies. The Health of the Nation A Strategy for Health in England (1992) and Scotland's Health A Challenge To Us All (1992) are strategies which identify secondary prevention as central planks of an approach which seeks to encourage a shift from a medical, sickness model of health care to a health promotion one (McKie *et al*, 1993).

In the Health of the Nation a target is set for the reduction:

> *"...in the incidence of invasive cervical cancer by at least 20% by the year 2000 (from a 1986 baseline)... The Government believes that the priority for this area must be the continued development*

of good practice in operating the screening programme, and in encouraging women to be screened. " (Dept of Health, 1992, p69)

The Scottish strategy does not set a specific target for a reduction in deaths due to cervical cancer but highlights the potentially preventable nature of the disease. The strategy does focus upon the implementation of the current screening programme (Scottish Office, 1992, p31).

At a local level the implications for nursing practice in primary health are evident; the provision of a screening service is not enough, this service must be actively used by 80% of the target population in a five year period and preferably attract those most at risk on a regular basis.

For women there are also many implications. Previous research has demonstrated that women experience embarrassment, fear and on some occasions pain when undergoing a smear test (Savage *et al*, 1989). In addition the need to meet targets may result in further time pressures on service organisation thus limiting the potential for women to seek and gain coherent and comprehensive information. Those women who are in the low risk group, such as the young woman who is not sexually active and the older woman who has had a hysterectomy, may be called for a test and experience unnecessary worry. The likelihood of cervical abnormalities amongst these groups is slim.

We began the design of our research project before the development of the GP contract and health strategies. However our work proved especially timely as these documents failed to address the specific question of what would encourage a women to take part in regular screening, rather than what would act as a barrier (Akehurst *et al*, 1991).

Researching Women's Health

Even those who do not yet believe that there can be an approach to research which can be justifiably called a feminist methodology have recognised the absence of a gender perspective in much of social research (Hammersley, 1992). Many feminist researchers have emphasised the necessity for a gender perspective in research in order to raise the visibility of women's experience (Ramazanoglu, 1992, Gelsthorpe, 1992).

Women have a special interest in knowing that health services are being monitored and evaluated as a matter of routine. They are more likely to be involved routinely with health issues in relation to their own reproductive cycles, and they are most likely to act on behalf of children over health matters.

An important issue addressed by many feminist researchers (Duelli Klein 1983; Mies 1983; Reinharz 1983) is the level to which the research is 'for' the women participants rather than 'about' or 'on' them (Roberts, 1992). This can be reflected in the way in which the data is collected, such as how much is explained about the study to the participants; how much they are offered the chance to use their own language and determine the direction of the enquiry. It may also determine whether participants are offered information about the results, or even invited to take part in the analysis and the writing up. Many of these are not possible, because of the time available for the study, or the requirements of the funding source, or because the participants do not wish to take up the offer, or are anonymous and so not contactable. However, if any or all are possible, they provide means by which the place and existence of the participants can be acknowledged, and so contribute to the visibility of women. Research can be designed, and questions can be asked, which either highlight the position of women, or deny it. Thus the form of the research design is often less important than what is taken for granted within the process of design.

The qualitative approach to research, discussed in earlier chapters, involves in-depth detail which is specific to each case, in the form of semi or unstructured interviews or field observations. These methods offer the opportunity for respondents to take the time to explore issues in a way they may not have had the chance to previously. In the case of cervical screening such an approach may be the only means of ensuring that women have the confidence to explore issues. This approach can allow complex, sensitive or embarrassing information to emerge, which frequently not only provides facts, but also explanations about how the facts came about. The limitations to this approach are that this kind of data collection is very time consuming, and consequently it is rare for a study to be able to use other than a small sample. Any claims made about the responses can only be made about the specific respondents, and cannot be generalised to a wider population. Because the enquiry is not a set of standard questions, the comparisons between what is said in terms of similarities and differences can only be the interpretation of the researcher, and cannot be tested statistically.

By contrast the quantitative approach involves standard questions taken to relatively large numbers of people who are selected randomly from the population in question. This may take the form of an interview schedule or questionnaire and may be completed by the respondent or an interviewer. Important characteristics of this approach are that the study can be replicated and generalised to the population from which the sample has been drawn. Each time the rules governing this approach are broken, or modified, any claims of the results are weakened. Nevertheless it is the quantitative approach which has characterised medical and much social research whilst qualitative research methods have been associated with feminist methodology and the attainment of a voice for the respondents. Not surprisingly these debates were evident in the negotiation of the research methods for the cervical screening project in which social researchers and medical practitioners had to debate the conduct of the project.

Origins of the Research Proposal

As with many research initiatives this one evolved as a result of a series of linked events and the on-going interests of certain individuals. These events involved the combination of:

1. Existing work on inequalities in health in the Northern Region area, conducted by a team of well known and highly regarded academics (Townsend, Philmore and Beattie, 1988)

2. Political controversy caused by the leaking of a paper from the Office of Population and Census Surveys which demonstrated a high incidence of positive smear tests in the Cleveland area

3. Structural support which was provided by the recently initiated Centre for Local Research (CLR) at Cleveland's institution for higher education, Teesside Polytechnic (now Teesside University)

These events came together in late 1987. The CLR had obtained a copy of the leaked document on the incidence of positive smear tests. This demonstrated an above average incidence of positive smears in economically deprived areas of Teesside. Academic staff working in the CLR invited local health service practitioners, planners and campaigners to a meeting to discuss the potential for a research agenda on health. Ten people attended, the majority of whom were health workers. Two of those attending had previously conducted research work on women's health for the local community health councils. On their suggestion it was agreed that health, and specifically women's health, required further research work conducted from a local perspective. Such suggestions were given added impetus by the work of the County social services who wished to conduct their own research into deprivation in certain wards of Cleveland. Local politicians in this Labour controlled area were also highlighting health as a national political issue.

Having agreed that work between 'town and gown' was both possible and desirable a series of meetings were set up to discuss a range of possible research questions. After several meetings it was clear that the issue of cervical screening was of interest to all parties probably fuelled by the controversy surrounding the leaked document. Researching cervical screening became the broad topic.

The next step was to decide on the research questions, methods and sources of funding. Again an event was to help focus attention. A local pathologist agreed to talk to the group about the process of reviewing slides of cervical cells. At this meeting several things became apparent, namely:

1. That information on patterns of take-up of smear tests was patchy

2. That the medical profession had only anecdotal evidence on the views of service users

3. Little was known, but a lot assumed, about the non-user of the service

Following a heated debate the following research aims were agreed:

1. To ascertain the pattern of take-up of cervical smear tests in the Cleveland area, namely the North Tees and South Tees District Health Authorities

2. To seek the attitudes of women residing in two deprived electoral wards concerning the smear test, the screening service and cervical cancer, whether or not they had experienced a smear test

Throughout the project women from ethnic communities were to be encouraged to participate. The research was to be located in both of the health districts and thus support was gained from health service management, practitioners and the County Council. From the inception of the group all were aware that funding would have to be secured. Whilst goodwill was evident it would not support the work of a researcher and research team to collect and analyse data. And it was now estimated that the work envisaged would take at least one year with nine months of that solely required for data collection. By mid 1988 several of the group, one academic and two health professionals, had written and submitted a proposal to the Economic and Social Research Council (ESRC). During this time we learnt the art of grant application, writing it on the run. None of us had completed such an application; we were ignorant of the time needed to do so. In addition we had little idea of what to cost and how to plan finances. But the support of the research group and ESRC staff was to prove invaluable. In the summer of 1988 we received the news that, much to our surprise, the application had been successful. Now we had the money to employ a full time researcher for nine months, a research team to administer the questionnaire survey and finance the analysis of the data. We had now commenced stage two of the research process.

A Practical Approach

One particularly lively debate held during the writing of the research proposal concerned the research methods that might be used. It was felt that the topic was too personal and the issues not predictable enough for a questionnaire survey to be adequate. It was important to allow women the opportunity to describe their feelings and experiences in their own words, and in a way that would encourage them to mention anything that they felt was relevant to this particular health service. To this end it was decided to use a series of small scale, taped, discussion groups to work through a series of issues related to the smear test experience. However the medical practitioners in the group were concerned that the discussion group work would not be considered as representative nor valid when it came to reporting our results. The discussion group method makes no pretence at providing data which might be analysed by statistics and thus generalisable to the population. It is a method which encourages in-depth response of feelings and beliefs; particularly important when ascertaining the views of those who had not used the screening service. Nevertheless a compromise was reached. It was agreed that a maximum of fifteen discussion groups would be conducted and after an initial analysis to be followed by the writing of a questionnaire which would be administered to women residing in two local authority estates.

National epidemiological data indicated that the incidence of positive smear tests was increasing in younger women and deaths were predominately occurring in the 50 plus age groups. It became important to target, at the questionnaire stage, the views of women aged 20 to 34 and women aged 50 to 64.

All the above debates were lengthy, at times heated, but ultimately we agreed a proposal which was strongly supported by all groups in the County and region. It was the hope of those who wrote the proposal that this support would ensure an ownership of the research by women respondents, the women of Cleveland and those designing and working in health services.

The overall results of this study are not generalisable. Nevertheless the project provides a mechanism for constructing a body of knowledge on a subject crucial to the lives of women and service provision.

Management of the Study

The final proposal involved a project which would take nine months for preparation, fieldwork and data collection, data processing and initial analysis, and a further six months for writing the report. The research assistant was appointed (one of the authors of this chapter) and began work in January of 1989. To complicate matters, the project director, the academic involved in writing the proposal (other author of this chapter) took up a new post at the University of Glasgow. As a consequence the researcher was working from home near Cleveland whilst the project director was teaching in Glasgow.

Ironically this situation proved to be useful in the management of the project. It certainly focused the need for communication between the director and full time researcher. Regular meetings took place once every six to eight weeks when the research assistant spent several days in Glasgow or the project director travelled down to the research site. In between we kept in telephone communication at least three times a week. Action plans were made at the regular meetings; feedback and modifications were made via the telephone links. On reflection we agreed that this formalisation of communication worked well, a routine was established which is not always used in projects in which director and researcher are working from the same department.

This long distance arrangement did, however, have an effect upon the involvement of the two other grant holders, who were located in different establishments. The level of their input to the design and day to day running of the project was reduced. And the wider research group ceased to meet. This was due in part to the move of the project director but also the belief that everyone would meet again on the completion of the cervical cancer data collection. Whilst we did all meet at the launch of the final project report in October 1990 the group that met and worked so hard in 1987 and 1988 lost impetus and died away.

The implications of how a project will be managed and conducted are rarely the first things to be considered at the design stage, or even during to course of the exercise. The immediacy of getting the project funded and then underway tended to take priority.

On reflection we have regrets at the falling off of communication but it tends to be those already heavily committed who take an interest in the developments noted above. Work commitments may be heavy and time limited. Thus the apparently natural division of labour — that the full time researcher and project director get on with the data collection and analysis whilst the consultative group provide support as requested - can result in ownership becoming focused upon the few rather than the many.

Design Decisions

As with many research projects, the proposal contained a basic research design, with an outline of the techniques to be used and the population to be sampled. Within that framework, decisions had to be made as the research progressed, about how and who should be sampled, what form the discussion groups should take, what questions should be asked in the second stage. The team defined criteria to enable the identification of appropriate geographical areas. A number of factors were considered. The County Cleveland Social Services Department was conducting a wider ranging health survey in the area and it was considered useful to select the areas to be used for our study from those used for this. This would allow comparisons to be made with the results, and possibly a sharing of contacts and techniques. However due to a delay in starting the local authority work the co-ordination did not take place.

Discussion Groups

The research team then went on to identify contacts in the community who would aid our access to the discussion groups we needed. This process can be complex and time consuming. Appropriately called the 'snowball' technique, it involves starting with a small number of possible contacts, using a range of communication approaches, such as writing, telephoning, visiting, and gradually building up a wider and wider range of contacts. Some will prove fruitful, meetings will be set up and discussion groups arranged and conducted. Some become *'cul de sacs'* very early on in the enquiry, but the most frustrating are those that seem promising until the very last moment, and then disappear. A discussion group may be set up, and no one turns up, or some other problem occurs.

It had been decided early on in our study to approach existing groups, rather that try to set up ad hoc groups just for the purpose of the study from the general public. This frequently solved the problem of the venue, and usually gave us a particular person, who was our first point of contact, who could introduce the researcher, and in some way validate her position. In the end nine groups were recruited in two electoral wards located either side of the river, that is, one in the Middlesborough area (North Tees District Health Authority) and one in the Stockton area (South Tees District Health Authority). The groups were quite diverse, some meeting regularly and in the form that we used, such as 'mother and toddler' groups, or an elderly persons luncheon club. Others met less frequently or took a different form just for our discussions, such as women members of a local residents group, or of a primary school parents group.

This method is not without its problems. The women participating were self selected and occasionally one or several women dominated a group discussion. In addition the negotiation of discussion depended upon the role of the researcher as a facilitator who attempted to achieve a balance in participation. Discussions lasted for up to two hours and were taped. Women were able to follow through stories in their own words and explore the attitudes of themselves and others. They also posed questions to each other and the researcher in a search for clarification of all aspects of the screening service and cervical cancer. The researcher found herself in some difficult situations as the medical knowledge of the research team was limited! Nevertheless, the research team were able to distribute relevant leaflets and provide information on further points of contact.

One major disappointment was the non-involvement of groups from ethnic communities. We began to realise that much more time would be needed to develop trust and a working relationship with these communities; in particular the Asian community. We applied to the ESRC for further funds to pursue this work, but we were informed by the ESRC that further monies would not be considered until data from the on-going project was analysed.

The discussion groups recruited provided a wide range of perspectives concerning health generally and the service itself, both within and between groups. This meant both background, such as age, marital and child care experiences, and the smear test experience itself. Our numbers were too small, and our sampling not systematic enough for us to be able to make firm claims that the experiences that our participants could be seen as representative of most women. It was, however, significant to the research team that, despite their many background differences, our participants reported many similarities in their beliefs about and the outcomes from using the service. Our selection of participants was not subject to the systematic chance of probability reflected in a randomly recruited group from a specified population. The nature of this stage of our study precluded that kind of approach. We needed to target specific people — women — living the area, who were relatively easy to locate, and were already involved in groups that we could contact.

The Questionnaire

The questionnaire stage of the study was in some ways more orderly, but in others more frustrating. The results of the discussions had to be translated into questions that would be asked in a far more formal manner. Ideas and views, sometimes complicated and not fully thought through, that had come out in the free flow of conversation and sharing, had to be structured in a way that was easy to understand and straightforward to answer. In order not to constrain the respondents too much, we constructed a questionnaire that continued to allow, where possible, the respondents to use their own words. The more straightforward factual questions used a multiple choice format, but questions about feelings and opinions were left open ended to allow some level of free expression.

We were very lucky to be able to employ the interview team of the Research and Development Department of Cleveland County Council. This team has a well established track record of conducting survey research. Thus the data collection for this stage was handed over to a team of experienced interviewers who were given a randomly selected set of three hundred respondents to be interviewed, one hundred and fifty in each of the two wards we were working in. This hand over took place at a training day, in which the researchers went through the questionnaire, question by question to ensure each was clearly understood. Again, the questionnaire had been tested out in a different geographical area with a small number of people to try to eliminate any misunderstandings.

Analysis of Discussion Group Data

Discussion group data was far from orderly. The format by which the discussion was conducted remained as open and flexible as possible. Although we had ideas about what the women might say, we could not assume that these might include everything, or indeed anything that they would consider relevant. We had designed a series of four themes to work through, leading from the general to the particular, which was intended to ensure that the discussion did not drift too far from the point. The themes distributed at meetings to women were:

1. What is meant by the term health?

2. How do you feel about your health?

3. What do you think of the smear test?

4. Comments on health service provision

We had tested it out with a set of groups in a different geographical location, to make sure that it worked. It was reassuring to discover that the themes that we devised, fitted in with the direction the women tended to go, although not always in the same order. Movement between the themes became fluid, flowing back and forth as ideas developed and crystallised.

This kind of data frequently results in a level of interpretation taking place in a way not found in a structured interview or questionnaire. Much of what the women had to say in discussion indicated similarities rather than differences, but they did not always use the same words to describe those similarities. The tapes were transcribed and themes awarded a code. Similar themes were drawn out across the discussion groups, and likewise differences.

Many of the women described feelings of embarrassment or fear and illustrated them with very different anecdotes, but the feelings were the same. With some of the women, not necessarily the most articulate, the feelings were very clear. They knew exactly what they approved of or disliked about their treatment. Others were unsure, uneasy, but less able to pinpoint what the problems were.

Analysis of Questionnaire Data

The responses from the questionnaires were less complex, but nevertheless required a considerable amount of post coding. Interpretations had to be made of all the open ended questions in order that a statistical analysis could be made. The women who agreed to take part had their own way of describing what it was like to have an internal examination, how they felt about it, what they understood to be a positive smear, or the treatment for cervical cancer. Thus the women's words had to be lost in an over-arching term which drew their different expressions into one meaning.

Upon coding 498 variables were designated, that is the number of personal characteristics, questions and categorised responses! The open ended nature of many of the questions resulted in this large number of variables. Analysis was conducted by the computer programme Statistics Package for Social Sciences (SPSS): frequencies and correlations (that is the measurement of the strength of a relationship between two variables) were calculated.

Dissemination

The funding body demanded, as all good funding bodies do, a written report within six months of completion of the project, and this formed the basis of our approach to dissemination. The format of the study, with it's two fairly discrete parts, allowed us to construct a set of chapters which addressed the different stages of the study, and which could then be developed into a series of articles that addressed different aspect of the study. The report was submitted to the ESRC in June 1990. Copies were provided to all interested parties who had contributed to the conception and the process of the project. Copies were also lodged with the Community Health Council Offices in Middlesborough, freely available to participants, interested researchers and planners. Newspaper articles were written by local and national journalists concerned with specific aspects of the study, and some unexpected by-products, have been published in a number of magazines and journals.

More important, however, was our obligation to the people who had made the study possible, especially the women who had given up their time and been so frank and open with their views and experiences. The research team had a commitment to acknowledge their invaluable contribution, and to offer them the opportunity to find out the results of the study. A public meeting was arranged for October 1990, to which all contributors and participants were invited. At that event the research team presented a selection of the most significant results, and were available for questions and further discussion.

It was hoped that the research would be taken further, especially in the area of service delivery and organisation and that the question of the views of women from ethnic communities would be addressed. Whilst the former did appear to occur and we were involved in GP and practice nurse training, the latter question of further research dwindled away due to a lack of funding and individuals in the locality willing to promote the issues.

Implications of the Research Process

Research, if nothing else, is a learning experience for all participants for a number of different reasons. If it works the way you want it to it provides a new and exciting viewpoint to an existing social phenomena, or it will confirm or reject existing theories or assumptions. It should contribute to a body of knowledge, provide new insights, point to new directions, and in some eyes, most importantly offer practical ideas which will inform and shape social policy and action. But research can have a number of other end products as well.

Our project, although small in both size and time scale, had effected the researchers, both on a personal level and in their understandings of the research process. It is perhaps easier to look back on a project to identify what issues concerning the research process have come up consistently. There is not normally the time to examine these kinds of issues during the course of a research project, when timetables and deadlines act as an imperative to action rather than reflection, and any speculation is reserved for the actual research results.

A Personal Learning Experience

The discussion groups had a particularly special impact upon us, as researchers, as we came into personal contact with the women during the discussions, and afterwards as we worked on the analysis of what the women felt about the smear test. It became very clear at a very early stage in the study that these women were not passive receivers of information and advice to which they either 'complied' or did not. These women lead busy demanding lives full of responsibilities, not just for themselves, but for members of their families, their homes, their jobs. As with most people, they had to prioritise their activities, with those that seemed the most urgent taking precedence. This service was used when an individual was symptom free, and more often than not operated with no communication taking place if the results were negative (i.e. desirable). Preventive methods of this kind have some difficulty overcoming the traditional medical model which discourages people from consulting their doctors unless they can identify clear symptoms to which a diagnosis may be attached. The smear test itself is at best uncomfortable, frequently painful and embarrassing, and carries some explanations that imply unacceptable sexual behaviour that many women would not consider applied to themselves. For these barriers to be overcome a sensitive approach is needed when explaining what the tests are for, why they are important, and how they are conducted. The conditions under which the tests are conducted, the attitudes of those involved with taking the test, will combine together with the effectiveness of the advice process to influence each woman as she decides whether and when she will use this kind of service. We, as researchers, collected our data — what the women had to say — and translated it into a report of what influence women's attitudes to the smear tests and made recommendations about how changes to the service could improve the take up rates. We, as women, recognised in ourselves similar feelings and experiences to those of the women. We found the discussions that took place influencing our own feelings and actions in connection with our own smear test decisions.

A Research Learning Experience

The research process involves a sequence of negotiations which frequently result in some level of compromise. The textbooks set out rules which govern the various research stages, from the initial design of the proposal to the analysis and interpretation, all of which provide recognised justifications for the claims that will be made about the research results. The research project introduces the painful reality of doing research and making decisions about the level to which it will be possible to conform to those rules.

In this particular project, compromises can be detected at the earliest stage, the proposal. The research team were committed to an approach which recognised the place of the subjects of the research in the project design. Methods which would allow the women's own words to be used was considered a priority. This would go some way towards acknowledging the invisibility of women in society, particularly in research, and contribute towards changing that position. A qualitative technique such as discussion groups was ideal for this purpose. Nevertheless, the preference of certain contributors for the use of quantitative methods resulted in the introduction of a second stage to the project involving a questionnaire to be taken to enough respondents to allow tests of statistical significance to be made. Time and access constraints resulted in four test discussion groups, and nine groups in the main project. The discussion groups were intended to inform the shape and content of the questionnaire. The questionnaire was intended to provide a quantitative confirmation of the theoretical constructs that emerged from the analysis of the discussions. However, the issues which arose in discussion emerged in a way that was both gradual and collective. The discussion was a process as well as a vehicle. To reconstruct the results as clear cut questions removes the process, and thus the method by which the answers can be reached. The inclusion of open-ended questions retained the chance for some individual processing to take place, but at the price of introducing yet another layer of analysis, that is, the post-coding process.

At the analysis stage there are always compromises — what to include, what to leave out. In qualitative analysis we must constantly monitor what is significant for us as individuals, even as researchers, which might influence the significance we attach to it in analytic terms. We look at our volumes of rich data, and meaningful quotes, and have to decide which truly represents the point we are trying to make. In our particular study we had a similar problem with our quantitative data. In attempting to do justice to what the women had said in the first stage, we had made our questionnaire very comprehensive. Although there were a number of issues that we felt we could not address directly, such as the issues around sexuality, and sexual relationships, we included a number of questions about the reproductive cycle, which had been raised explicitly in the discussions, or might allow women to mention sexuality issues if they wanted to do so. Although not directly related to the smear test, or to cervical cancer, these matter were raised frequently enough for us to feel that they were related in some way. Whether the women who were asked these questions would understand these issues in the same way as the women in the discussions could not be certain, because the process by which they constructed their replies could not be recorded. It was reassuring to find, therefore, that where comparisons could be made between the results of the two stages, there were strong similarities. Again time and resources intervened and only a proportion of the potential analysis of the questionnaire could be attempted. The report addressed the main questions identified in the research design, that is: what are the attitudes of women towards the cervical smear test, as reflected in their views and experiences. The fact that their views are influenced by their gender roles, their family lives, their social interaction could only be touched upon in the analysis and the reporting.

These compromises do not undermine the results or the claims made by the researchers. Provided that they are recognised by the researcher during the research process, they can actually contribute to the validity of the exercise by acting as a very subjective act of reflexivity, constantly reminding the researcher of her place in the exercise, and her views in the process. Personal preference and accidental bias can creep into research at any stage. Most people chose their research topics because of a personal interest, which can fire enthusiasm, and point direction. But subjectivity does not have to be an uncontrollable urge that weakens the process and damages the results. If acknowledged and monitored it can make a valuable contribution to understanding and interpretation.

Postscript

From 1990 we have continued to analyse and present the results of the project. Copies of the final report were requested by individuals and groups from throughout the UK and Europe. Local services did amend leaflets describing the service and cervical cancer . We participated in local training for GPs and practice nurses as well as writing papers for academic audiences. Most pleasing, perhaps, was the recognition the discussion group method received from health professionals and local groups. Unfortunately further work, especially work with women from ethnic communities, has not taken place. As key individuals left the locality or changed jobs the research seemed to become a product of a particular time and combination of people.

Acknowledgements

The authors would like to acknowledge the invaluable support and input of:

- the women of Cleveland
- Dr Tony Garrett, North Tees District Health Authority and Ms Irene Bellerby, South Tees District Health Authority
- the staff of the screening and cytology service in both North and South Tees
- the staff of North Tees Community Health Council

The authors would also like to acknowledge the support of the

ESRC grant number R000231171.

References

Central Statistical Office (1992) *Social Trends*. HMSO, London

Chamberlain J (1984) Failure of the Cervical Cytology Screening Programme. *Br Med J*, **289**, 853–54

Chomet J and Chomet J (1989) *Cervical Cancer*, Grapewine Press, Wellingborough

Day N (1989) Screening for Cancer of the Cervix. *J Epidem Comm Health*, **43**, 103–6

Dean K (1992) Double burdens of work: the female work and health paradox. *Health Prom Intl*, **7**(1), 17–25

Department of Health and Social Security (1988) *Health Services Management: Cervical Cancer Screening* (HC(88)1). DHSS, London

Department of Health (1989) *General Practice in the NHS: A New Contract*. DoH, London

Department of Health (1992) *The Health of the Nation A Strategy for Health in England*, DoH, London

Gregory S and McKie L (1992) Researching Cervical Cancer: Compromises, practices and beliefs. *J Adv Health Nurs Care*, **2**(1), 73–84

Gelsthorpe L (1992) 'Response to Martyn Hammersley's paper 'on feminist methodology'. *Sociol* **26**(2): 213–18

Hammersley M (1992) 'On Feminist Methodology'. *Sociol* **26**(2): 187–206

Duelli Klein R (1983) 'How to do what we want to do: thoughts about feminist Methodology'. In: Bowles G and Duelli Klein R (eds), *Theories of Women's Studies*. Routledge & Kegan Paul, London

McKie L, Gregory S (1992) Women's Health: Policy and Practice, *J Adv Health Nurs Care* **2**(1): 59–60

McKie L (1993a) Women's Views of the Cervical Smear Test: Implications for Nursing Practice — Women who have not had a Smear Test. *J Adv Nurs* **18**: 972–79

McKie L (1993b) Women's Views of the Cervical Smear Test: Implications for Nursing Practice — Women who have had a Smear Test. *J Adv Nurs* **18**: 1228–34

Mies M (1983) 'Towards a methodology for feminist research'. In: Bowles G and Duelli Klein R eds. *Theories of Women's Studies.* Routledge & Kegan Paul, London

Morgan D (1990) 'Men, Masculinity and the process of sociological enquiry'. In: Roberts H ed. *Doing Feminist Research.* Routledge and Kegan Paul, London

Oakley, A (1981) 'Interviewing Women: A Contradiction in Terms' In: Roberts H ed. *Doing Feminist Research.* Routledge and Kegan Paul, London

Posner T (1993) Ethical Issues and the Individual Woman in Cancer Screening Programmes. *J Adv Health Nurs Care*, **2**(3): ****

Ramazanoglu C (1992) 'On feminist methodology:male reason versus female empowerment' *Sociol* **26**(2): 207–12

Reinharz, S (1983) Experiential analysis: a contribution to feminist research. In: Bowles G and Duelli Klein R eds. *Theories of Women's Studies.* Routledge & Kegan Paul, London

Roberts H (1981) *Doing Feminist Research.* Routledge & Kegan Paul, London

Roberts H (1981) Women and their doctors: power and powerlessness in the research process. In: Roberts H ed. *Doing Feminist Research.* Routledge and Kegan Paul, London

Roberts H (1985) '*The Patient Patients: Women and their Doctors'* Pandora, London

Roberts H (1992) '*Women's Health Matters'* Routledge. London

Savage W, Schwarz M and George J (1989) *A Survey of Women's Knowledge, Attitudes and Experience of Cervical Screening in the Tower Hamlets Health District.* The London Hospital, Whitechapel, London

Scottish Office (1992) *Scotland's Health A Challenge To Us All.* Scottish Office, Edinburgh

Townsend P, Philmore P and Beattie A (1988) *Health and Deprivation.*

Inequality and the North. Croom Helm, New York

Whitehead M (1987) *The Health Divide: Inequalities in Health in the 1980s,* Health Education Council, London

CHAPTER 9
RESEARCHING CERVICAL SCREENING SERVICES

Tina Posner

This chapter discusses differences of method and aspects of process, and the results produced in two UK research projects in which the author was involved investigating women's views of cervical screening and its consequences. The first project involved large scale population surveys analysed by the SPSS computer programme, the second was an in-depth study of the experiences of a series of women going through a medical process; both were funded by the Cancer Research Campaign.

The first project to be discussed grew out of negotiations between the director (who designed the protocol and was based elsewhere) and the health educator involved. The author was employed as the research officer to execute the project. Two surveys were carried out on a random sample of the female population[1] as part of the evaluation of a programme of 'education and persuasion' in relation to cervical screening[2] before (1979) and after (1981), the

---

1   *This sample was selected from the Electoral Register and is likely to have somewhat under-represented younger women.*

2   *The project had the title `The evaluation of education and persuasion related to screening for cervical cancer in high-risk populations'. Directed by Dr P Hobbs from the Dept of Epidemiology and Social Research at the University of Manchester, it was carried out in Oxford by the author who was the research officer on the project with the help of a research assistant and temporary interviewers. The views expressed in this chapter, and any errors or omissions, are attributable to the author alone. Papers were presented by the author to the Annual Scientific Meeting of the Society for Social Medicine, 1981: 'Women's View of the Benefits of the Cervical Smear Test'; and The*

intervention programme. The first survey provided a baseline from which to assess the views of the women who took part in the programme; the second was a check for any major shifts of opinion which might have occurred in the intervening two years and an attempt to assess any 'ripple' effect from the programme. Together, the surveys were a fairly comprehensive study of women's experiences of screening and beliefs about cervical cancer, with 680 women interviewed on the first survey, and 700 on the second. At that time, a common assumption among people working in the field of health 'education' was that 'fear and ignorance' were the reasons why some women did not attend for a cervical smear test.

Discovering a lay/medical difference of view

One of the questions on the first survey was an open-ended question designed to investigate women's view of the benefit of the test. Previously, the focus had been on efforts to get across a message about the unquestioned medical view of the benefit; prevention of the development of cervical cancer through detection of early neoplastic changes, and women's view of the benefit had not been sought. The question asked 'What would you say was the main benefit of the cervical smear test?' The interviewers were instructed to record the answers verbatim and these were subsequently submitted for content analysis. As this question followed questions about their own experiences, but preceded questions about the curability and detectability of cervical cancer, and was entirely open with no prompting, there was reason to assume that the range of answers was a good reflection of the pattern of women's views of the benefit of having the test. In their enthusiasm for breaking new

---

British Sociological Association Medical Sociology Annual Conference, 1982: `Women's Beliefs about Cervical Cancer'.

ground and not making assumptions about how women thought, the researchers, who were new to survey research, overlooked the problem of categorising 680 answers so that the data could be included in the computer analysis.

The analysis of the answers resulted in the identification of five basic answer components; reassurance, early detection, diagnosis, prevention and ambiguity. (Answers were categorised according to their components rather than giving precedence to one component over another). The results demonstrated that the prime benefit of having the test from a woman's point of view, was the reassurance and peace of mind that comes from knowing she is 'all right'. As table 1 shows, reassurance was the most often mentioned benefit (by 42%), and prevention the least often mentioned (by 4%). Women who had had a test were more likely to mention reassurance and early detection as benefits ($p < .0001$); women who had never been tested were more likely to be ambiguous about the benefits ($p < .0001$).

Table 9.1: Cervical smear benefits components:

Untested/tested women

Answer component	Totals n = 680	Untested n = 241	Tested n = 439	Statistical significance
	%	%	%	
Reassurance	42	14	57	$p < 0.0001$
Early detection	21	15	26	$p < 0.0001$
Diagnosis	17	16	18	n.s.
Prevention	4	3	4	n.s.
Ambiguous	13	27	5	$p < 0.0001$

Survey findings deny ignorance

Women's generally optimistic attitudes towards the curability and detectability of cervical cancer were shown by their answers to a set of questions included in both surveys. These asked whether they thought cervical cancer was curable, whether they thought it was detectable at an early stage and whether they thought early treatment increased the chance of cure or made no difference. Around 80% thought cervical cancer was curable, 84% that it was detectable at an early stage, and nearly 90% that early treatment increased the chance of cure. We do not know to what extent the high degree of optimism found was due to knowledge that there is a high rate of cure of cervical cancer in particular, or to an increased optimism about cancer in general. However, it was clear that with such high rates of belief in the early detectability and curability of cervical cancer and the advantage of early treatment, ignorance about the medical benefits of screening could no longer be assumed to be the reason for failure to attend.

A question in the first survey asked '*Some women don't want to have the test done at all. Have you any idea why that might be?*' Analysis of the answers found that nearly half the respondents suggested fear, anxiety or worry as a reason, and that women in the age groups most likely to have had a test, most often mentioned fear and embarrassment. The answers to this question appeared to reflect common negative feelings about the test, with anxiety and embarrassment being to some extent, part of many women's experience of the test.

Protective measures

Women's beliefs about ways to protect themselves from cervical cancer were investigated by different means on the two surveys. The first survey included an open-ended question: 'Do you know if there is anything a woman can do to avoid getting cancer of the cervix (the neck of the womb)?' In the second survey, there was a question which presented statements about possible ways to protect oneself from cervical cancer, with which the respondents were asked to agree or disagree. The statements were based on suggestions made in answer to open-ended questions[3] in the earlier survey. A wide discrepancy was found between the responses to the open-ended question and to the statements.

Just over a third (36%) of the women interviewed on the first survey replied with a suggestion of something a woman could do to avoid getting cancer of the cervix. Additionally, 4% of the respondents, objecting to the implication that cervical cancer was preventable, said either that there was '*nothing you can do to avoid it*' or '*...to prevent it*', but you could have a cervical smear test to detect it early, or replied simply '*don't know apart from...*' and then mentioned the cervical smear test. The answers to this question were subjected to content analysis which produced five main answer categories; medical check-ups, hygiene measures, relating to sexual intercourse, relating to contraception and vaginal irritants, and a group of more general factors. Most of those who suggested medical check-ups as a way to avoid getting cervical cancer (36%), specifically mentioned the cervical smear test (32%). Of those, 11% who mentioned hygiene measures, 9% talked of washing or being careful about personal hygiene. Five percent talked of avoiding certain types of sexual activity, particularly 'promiscuity', a few mentioning the avoidance of intercourse at an early age, or during menstruation, or 'too much intercourse'. A small proportion (2%), mentioned barrier methods of contraception, not taking the pill, and avoidance of talcum powder and other vaginal irritants. A

---

3   *Open-ended questions on the first survey included a question intended to tap lay beliefs about the aetiology of cervical cancer and its precursors: 'Do you know of anything which makes a woman more likely to develop cervical cancer?'*

similar proportion mentioned not smoking, having a good diet and other general health factors.

In the later survey, the question which asked women to agree or disagree with statements about possible ways of protecting themselves from cervical cancer had the following preamble:

I am going to read you some statements women have made about ways of protecting themselves from cancer of the neck of the womb, the cervix.

Only 12% disagreed with the first statement 'Women should be careful about personal hygiene'. The high proportion agreeing (79%) contrasts with the much smaller numbers (11%) spontaneously mentioning hygiene as a way to avoid getting cervical cancer in the earlier survey. Even though the preamble to the question said that the statements were about ways to protect oneself from cervical cancer, it may well be that much of the agreement was with the suggestion that hygiene is an important aspect of taking care of one's health, and the response cannot be taken as widespread belief that washing will protect women from getting cervical cancer. It seems likely that the answers to the open-ended question probably gave a truer picture of the proportion for whom the idea that washing could in some way be protective, was valid.

The response to the statement 'Woman who start having sex in their early teens are more likely to get cancer of the neck of the womb', was more evenly spread with 42% agreeing, 24% disagreeing and 34% undecided. There was considerable agreement with the statement 'Women who have sex with lots of men are more likely to get cancer of the neck of the womb', with over half the sample (56%) agreeing, 29% undecided and 15% disagreeing. These responses again contrast sharply with the 5% spontaneously mentioning some aspect of sexual activity in answer to the question on the earlier survey. It seems highly unlikely that the difference between the percentages can be accounted for by any increased media coverage of theories linking women's sexual behaviour with the aetiology of cervical cancer in the intervening two years. It is more likely that the form of the questions was the prime cause of the difference. Whereas the uncertainty and speculation surrounding the subject led interviewees to be hesitant to make suggestions in answer to the open-ended question, statements authoritatively read out from survey schedules lent credence to suspicion and half-recalled magazine articles, and agreement cannot be taken as a direct reflection of firmly held beliefs.

Asked to endorse the next statement 'Women should have a smear test regularly as a way of protecting themselves from cervical cancer', only 3% of the survey sample **disagreed**, though it was not clear whether they were adverse to the idea of the test altogether, or to regular screening. A small percentage (5%) were undecided, and there were qualifications such as 'it's up to the person concerned', 'if they feel they need it', 'if something's wrong' and 'it depends on age'. With such widespread agreement with the suggestion that cervical screening was protective, the health promotion task was not so much to persuade women that the test was a good thing, as to persuade all sections of the at-risk population that it had a function as a regular preventive check-up. This was further evidence that failure to take part in the cervical screening programme could not simply be ascribed to lack of awareness of the population benefits.

The response to the following three statements about different forms of contraception was unwillingness to be committed to either agreement or disagreement, with the undecided proportion the largest. A third of the survey responders disagreed with each of the statements: 'use a dutch cap (diaphragm) in family planning as a way of protecting oneself from cervical cancer', 'use a condom (sheath) ...', 'avoid using the pill ...'. The hesitancy to agree or disagree with statements on contraception was possibly a reflection of a belief that different types of contraception suit different women and thus general pronouncements are to be avoided. The preamble to the statements was some time away by then, and the interviewers may not always have repeated ˋas a way of protecting oneself from cervical cancer'. It seems also likely that the evidence that barrier methods of contraception could be protective (Richardson and Lyon, 1981) had not been publicised in the general population at that time.

Age group differences

There were important differences between women of different age groups in their responses to the above questions. These differences reflected both their different experiences in relation to cervical screening and their different beliefs, demonstrating cultural shifts over time.

A woman's view of the benefit of the cervical smear test was related to whether she herself had ever been screened, and this in turn was related to her age. Women in the older age group (55 and over) who were less likely to have had a test, were more likely to talk in ambiguous terms about the benefits, particularly if they thought it did not apply to them[4]. Women under 55 years were more likely than older women to mention reassurance as a benefit of the test. They were also more likely to think that cervical cancer was detectable at an early stage and curable, to mention the smear test as a protection against cervical cancer and to have actually had a test. These findings suggested a network of interrelated beliefs and motivations associated with a woman's age and the cervical smear test, and specifically, that relationships between belief in the early detectability of cervical cancer and the protective function of the

---

4   *It was found that older women in particular often thought the test was not applicable to them for one reason or another, the most common being that they were 'too old' for the test, that they had nothing wrong — no gynaecological symptoms, and therefore did not need it, or that they were unlikely to have 'that sort of trouble'. Some women thought that the test was no longer relevant if they were post-menopausal or if they had been widowed.*

by *Tina Posner*

test, and the perception of reassurance as a benefit, were mediated by age and reinforced by experience of the test.

Understandably, the women most likely to mention the cervical smear test spontaneously were those most likely to have actually had a test in the age group 35–54 years. The differences between the age groups in the proportions agreeing with the statement that women should have a cervical smear test regularly as a way of protecting themselves from cervical cancer, reflects the likelihood of women in that age group actually having had a test (p < .001, Table 2). Although the majority (85%) of women in the oldest age group (55–92 years), agreed with the idea of cervical screening, there was a large discrepancy in this group between those agreeing with the statement and those who had actually been screened (44%). Seventy-four percent of those disagreeing with the statement were in the older age group, and most of the qualifications about applicability were made by women in this group[4]. In the other two age groups, 95% agreed with the statement, with a small discrepancy between that proportion and the proportion who had been screened in the 35–54 age group (89%) and a rather larger discrepancy in the younger age group (18–34 years), 76% of whom had been screened. Some of the respondents in the older age group would already have been too old by the time cervical screening was introduced, and some in the youngest group would not yet have been old enough to have fallen into the population to be screened according to the policy at the time[5].

The idea that attention to personal hygiene could be protective against cervical cancer was evidently more prevalent amongst older women, with the proportion spontaneously

---

5   *The official screening programme at that time targeted sexually active women aged 35–64 years, and women under 35 years who had had three or more children. However, many younger women were screened at the suggestion of the family planning clinic or their GP, or at their own request.*

mentioning it increasing from 5% in the youngest to 16% in the oldest age group (p. < 001). Twice the proportion (47%) in the oldest age group agreed with the statement 'Women should be careful about personal hygiene as a way of protecting themselves from cancer of the neck of the womb' as in the 35-54 age group (23%). Agreement with the suggestions that 'women who start having sex ...early ...' and 'women who have sex with lots of men...' are more likely to get cervical cancer, increased with age. In the youngest age group, 38% **disagreed** with the first statement, but in the oldest the proportion disagreeing was only 14%. In relation to the statements about contraception, there was less disagreement and more uncertainty amongst women in the oldest age group as compared with the other two groups.

Table 9.2: Agreement that regular cervical screening is protective, according to age and whether tested

Age Group	Agree	Undecided	Disagree	Had test
	%	%	%	%
18–34	95	4.5	0.5	76
35–54	95	3.0	2.0	89
55–92	85	9.0	6.0	44

The survey findings demonstrated large differences between responses to open-ended and closed questions using statements about suggested actions, in an area rife with speculative theory. The survey results also showed the importance in this context of investigating age group differences, because of the differing experiences of the older and younger women and shifts over time in beliefs. The finding that there was widespread knowledge of the curability and early detectability of cervical cancer, and strong support for the cervical screening programme in general, was important feedback for the intervention programme, and implied that some previous assumptions about non-attendance for screening needed to be questioned.

Looking at the experience of a positive cervical smear result

Interviewing women about their experiences of cervical screening and discussions with the local consultant cytologist made this chapter's author aware of the considerable anxiety accompanying an abnormal cervical smear result. Patients undergoing treatment for cervical cancer had been the subject of some research attention but in the early 1980s almost no account had been taken of the position of well women found to have abnormal cervical cells as a result of taking part in the cervical screening programme. The success of the treatment of cervical intra-epithelial neoplasia (CIN) has been judged simply in terms of success in eliminating the abnormal cells. The impact of the medical process after a positive cervical smear had not been investigated, and the possibility of unnecessary morbidity in terms of physical, psychosocial or psychosexual distress resulting from medical intervention had been largely overlooked. Medical personnel involved — gynaecologists, colposcopists, nurses and GPs, recognised this omission and gave the research project[6] which was proposed, support and encouragement. It was also recognised within the funding organisation that this situation needed investigation. However, the attitude of the funding organisation's gatekeeper at the outset of the

---

6   *This project had the title 'Impact on patients of the medical process following discovery of an abnormal cervical smear'. It was carried out by the author while funded by the Cancer Research Campaign, with the support of Professor Martin Vessey while based in the Dept of Community Medicine and General Practice, University of Oxford between 1982 and 1985.*

research was that 'this is only a small problem'. It was not clear whether the problem was seen as small in terms of numbers of affected or in terms of the degree of possible distress involved. A problem which has not been widely recognised, articulated and discussed, may well not yet be on any agendas, and is unlikely to be seen as significant.

Women approached with an invitation to take part in the study[7], quickly understood that the focus of the enquiry was on their own experiences and enthusiastically endorsed the aim of the investigation. The timing of the interviews was designed to follow women through the process of medical intervention after a positive cervical smear finding, with 153 women attending two different hospitals, being interviewed two or three times (altogether 357 interviews). The initial interview was carried out in the out-patient department either just before or immediately after the colposcopy examination, the last interview approximately six months after the first, usually in the woman's home. The interviewees clearly welcomed the opportunity to talk about what was happening to them, and would, on occasion, make unscheduled visits to the room where interviews were conducted in the outpatient department, in order to keep the researcher informed about developments. This led to a sense of solidarity between researcher and researched which encouraged the researcher in her subsequent efforts to record and publicise the results of the investigation.

Taking part in the interviews would inevitably have had some effect on women's experience of the process being studied.

---

7   *Only one woman declined to take part in the study at all. She was an eighteen-year-old whose mother came in the interview room with her. It is possible that she was apprehensive about the questions she might be asked in her mother's presence. Four study participants did not want to be interviewed further at the post treatment stage, one woman saying and the others implying, that they 'had had enough of the whole business'.*

The opportunity to talk about a stressful situation with someone ready to listen and understand, can in itself be therapeutic. To have someone show interest in one's own reactions and thoughts and progress through a medical episode, can be affirming and is unlikely to have a detrimental effect. Recognition of this helped the researcher to overcome anxieties about recording others' distress without being in a position to do anything immediately to alleviate it. The investigation was attempting to describe and analyse the nature of any distress rather than 'measure' it in some way, and any beneficial effect of taking part in the research did not interfere with this aim. There were two situations in which the researcher felt she should intervene in a distinct way by giving the interviewee information which she would appear to need. In the first interview, when a woman was shortly to have a colposcopy examination but was totally lacking any information about the nature of the examination, the researcher gave a brief explanation at the end of the interview[8]. There were a few women who spoke in the last interview as if they had had cancer, when the condition for which they had been treated was clearly not found to be malignant[9]. The researcher would then take time at the end of the interview to provide an explanation of CIN for the interviewee to take (or leave) as she wished.

The semi-structured interviews were designed to provide both factual information and a record of the interviewees' thoughts and feelings about the medical process at different stages. The

---

8   *Nearly half the women interviewed in this study had no prior explanation of the colposcopy examination procedure. Having very little idea what to expect increased their anxiety about the uncertain implications of the abnormal smear findings. Some women thought that treatment could take place there and then, and one or two had come without having had breakfast in case they might need a general anaesthetic.*

9   *Any suspicion of invasive cancer was managed by a cone biopsy operation followed by a hysterectomy if the malignancy was confirmed.*

interviews included many open-ended questions to which the researcher recorded the results more or less verbatim. Clearly, it was important not to suggest ways of reacting to, or conceptualising what was going on, and not to 'put words into the mouths' of interviewees. However, this presented some methodological difficulties since there was a sense in which the interviewees did not possess the information and language for thinking about and thus talking about their (medical) condition — and this in itself was problematic. This did not mean there was any difficulty about articulating the 'human' condition in which they found themselves — as the whole study testified. Words used in the construction of questions were those which would already have been part of any medical or administrative communication with the women, such as 'abnormal cells' or 'positive smear' and 'colposcopy examination'. However, even using the word 'colposcopy', a word unfamiliar to most people, tended to change the status of the word from unknown and unpronounceable, to known and pronounceable, and thus part of a vocabulary. There was a need for particular care in the pre-colposcopy interview to avoid using words which might indicate a diagnosis. The word 'cancer' was used only if an interviewee had herself used it, in a question which asked: '*You mentioned your worry about the possibility of cancer. Has anyone you know, or anyone in your family had cancer?*' Mostly the questions asked what had been said about the condition. The interviews revealed a lay view of the investigation and outpatient treatment of CIN which differed significantly from the medical view that it was an 'essentially nonmorbid', minor procedure (Richard *et al*, 1980).

Discovering the cervix has feelings

It was accepted knowledge, handed down unquestioned from one generation of gynaecology students to another, that the uterine cervix was fairly insensitive. The explanation given was that there were 'few nerve endings'. The implication was that various medical procedures could be carried out on the cervix without the need to take account of the woman's feelings since she would be unlikely to feel very much. Any patient who complained of discomfort could be assumed to be abnormal in her sensitivity. This belief fitted in with the general assumption that the intervention caused no harm, and was sustained even though there was some evidence to the contrary.

The study gathered data on symptoms experienced by women undergoing the investigation and treatment. It soon became clear that the insensitivity of the cervix was a myth, some women experiencing acute discomfort. However, women varied considerably in what they felt, as colposcopists had often noted. Systematic documentation of their experiences both during the procedure in the clinic and afterwards, produced evidence that the treatment caused severe distress at the time to 42–44% (cryocautery/laser treatment) of patients, that this was more likely in nulliparous women ($p < 0.01$), and that some patients (30%) continued to suffer pain after the treatment was finished. A small percentage (8%) of women found the investigation itself (the colposcopy examination), 'painful', rather than merely uncomfortable (41%).

The wording of the questions may have been important in uncovering distress which could not be described simply in terms of physical pain. After colposcopy, interviewees were asked whether they had found the examination 'painful', as well as how they felt about the examination. After treatment, interviewees were asked whether the treatment 'hurt', how they felt afterwards and whether they had any symptoms afterwards. There was no attempt to quantify the degree of any discomfort, but an assessment of whether the distress experienced was severe was made according to the words used by the interviewee. A wider focus on the distress experienced allowed an analysis of other factors in the situation which could have contributed to making the treatment an ordeal for some patients. Women commented on their vulnerability and sense of exposure in the lithotomy position required for treatment, these feelings being heightened by the presence of observers or by any intrusion into the clinic. When they needed to be in this position for some length of time (ten to twenty minutes with cryocautery), physical and emotional discomfort could become acute[10].

A set of questions investigated women's experiences in the period after treatment and this uncovered distress and continuing symptoms which had not previously been taken into account and were important aspects of a woman's total experience of the medical intervention. Just over a quarter (26%) of the women reported that they were emotionally upset or depressed in the days shortly after treatment, feeling 'shaken', 'battered', 'weepy', 'delicate'. In order to try to minimise any negative impact of the treatment, it would be necessary to anticipate that some women could experience a degree of shock and traumatisation, and recommendations were made accordingly. Some women (30%) who underwent cryocautery complained of the heaviness and duration of the subsequent watery discharge. This could last for three or even four weeks, and could be very heavy in the first few days, so that frequent changes of sanitary towels were needed in order not to feel wet all the time. Cryocautery patients had not been warned to expect this 'physical mess' after treatment because it was not realised how extensive this could be.

Discovering the person behind the cervix

Nowhere was the need to take account of the person whose genital

---

10   *Resultant recommendations were that: observers should not be allowed into the colposcopy clinic unless it was absolutely necessary, and then only with the patient's consent; the clinic door should be locked during examination or treatment to prevent intrusions; care should be taken to ensure that the patient was made as comfortable as possible in this position.*

part was the subject of medical attention more evident than in the area of sexual relations. Here, the person's own history and psyche, in combination with the medical and societal presentation of the condition, affected how it was experienced.

This study revealed that the abnormal smear finding and subsequent medical process had a considerable psychosexual impact, with 43% of women saying that it had disturbed their sexual relations, and 14% that their sex life was not back to normal at the end of the process. This disturbance was in addition to the post-treatment interruption which was the subject of varying recommendations for abstention from sexual intercourse — two to six weeks according to different medical personnel. On first learning that they had an abnormal smear, some women were anxious about continuing to have sexual intercourse for fear that it would make their cervical condition worse, or that it could be transmitted to their partner. Since they might wait many weeks before seeing the colposcopist for further examination and discussion of their condition, they needed an earlier opportunity to talk about their anxieties. The GP or FPC doctor who initially explained the abnormal smear finding was the obvious person to do this, but only one woman mentioned having been reassured at this point. Contraceptive changes, co-existing symptoms and sexually transmitted disease, particularly HPV (genital warts), were additional causes of anxiety. However, an opportunity to discuss concerns in the area of sexual relations was very seldom provided by the clinic doctors. The possible need for counselling in this area of life, so obviously relevant to cervical abnormalities, had been ignored.

There was a notable disparity between this lack of attention and the amount of attention given in the media at the time to speculation about possible behavioural causes of cervical cancer and its precursors. The result of suggested links in the media between 'promiscuity' and the development of cervical cancer or CIN, was that women in the study tended to feel embarrassment about their condition, and some clearly felt stigmatised by the implied guilt:

'I felt dirty because of the documentary on TV ... talking about the permissive society and cervical cancer reaching epidemic proportions. I was worried that everybody would think I'd been sleeping with everybody.' (Posner and Vessey, 1988: 67)

Thus, not only was there a need for timely and accurate information and open discussion of issues, but also a need to heal the possible hurtfulness to a woman's sense of moral and personal integrity. Instead, patients at one of the hospitals were systematically questioned during history taking about the age at which they first had intercourse — the only medical question which provoked any complaints to the researcher because of its intrusive nature and lack of immediate clinical relevance.

Experiencing prevention

This study indicated that the episode was, generally, conceived and experienced within the curative rather than the preventive medical mode. To women going through the process, it felt as if cervical screening had found 'something wrong' which needed to be 'put right'. Rather than providing reassurance that all was well, the cervical smear test had resulted for them in a period of uncertainty and anxiety, about the nature and implications of the problem, and what the investigation and treatment involved. The greatest anxiety was experienced prior to the colposcopy investigation and while waiting to have treatment. After any initial alarm about cancer had been quelled, there remained concern about an ill-defined abnormality which was still medically significant enough to require treatment, though it was causing no symptoms and, they were assured, was no immediate threat to their wellbeing. The most common explanation in terms of 'abnormal cells', variously described, left the condition still vaguely defined. This was underscored perhaps when, having asked if the colposcopist explained what was found on the abnormal smear, the researcher asked if the colposcopist 'gave it a name'. Only in a few cases had an appropriate medical term been supplied by a colposcopist, and in the absence of a word, other than cancer (or pre-cancer), by which to refer to the condition, some women made comments such as (Posner and Vessey, 1988: 81):

I don't know what the problem's called. I haven't got a name for it.

I still don't know what the hell it was ... They involve you with it, but you don't know what you've been involved with.

She was very good. She was sat at the end of the bed. Came straight to the point ... I would have liked her to have said what was wrong.

In the grey area which was not cancer, but at the same time, not 'normal' and acceptable as far as medical judgement was concerned, there was, it became clear, a problem of conceptualisation. How the condition was thought about would clearly affect how it was experienced.

Nearly all the women in the study were well women who were treated for CIN, a condition which, depending on its severity, could reverse in a proportion of cases[11] without medical intervention, but is a risk factor for carcinoma of the cervix if left untreated. Removing the abnormal cells removes the risk, but the exact point where prevention becomes cure is blurred. One woman's explanation of her state — *'You feel as though you're ill and you're not'*, expressed the ambivalence of this condition. What was experienced was the threat, if not the actuality, of cancer. The study revealed that the mere suggestion of the possibility of cancer could carry the same negative metaphorical image as the fully developed disease, and this image tended to affect how a woman felt about her

---

11   *Estimates of the proportion of cases of CIN reversing spontaneously vary and depend on the degree of abnormality — anything between half and two-thirds of cases of CIN1 (mild abnormality) or CIN2 (moderate abnormality).*

body, her health status and her future prospects.

In the last (post-treatment) interview, beliefs about cancer in general and cervical cancer in particular were investigated. Although the large majority of women in the study (92%) thought that cervical cancer was curable if detected early or 'usually', for many (68%) their general view of cancer as a disease was still very negative, and equated with unstoppable bodily destruction and painful death. The domination of this prevailing cultural image of cancer in the absence of a more developed conceptualisation of CIN, meant that there was an ambivalent response to questions about future prospects — 63% of the interviewees could not feel confident that recurrence was unlikely, and over half (55%) continued to feel threatened by the possibility of cancer. Thus prevention could leave a woman feeling more vulnerable than before, and was certainly not painless, many women having physical symptoms as a result of treatment, besides psychosocial distress.

To invite an assessment of the overall impact and significance of the medical intervention, a question was devised using phrases previously used by interviewees. It asked *'Would you say that the investigation and treatment you've needed after the abnormal smear finding has been:*

- A bit of a nuisance but not much more

- A big upset and disruption in life

- Something you haven't really got over

- Something you've already largely forgotten about

It soon became clear that for most interviewees neither of the first two phrases felt quite right; the tenor of the first phrase was too dismissive of the episode and the word 'nuisance' considered inappropriate, but for most interviewees looking back, the episode, while upsetting, had not involved a big disruption of their life. A number of other words such as 'necessary', 'inconvenient', 'uncomfortable', 'unpleasant' were suggested in place of 'nuisance'. Most interviewees endorsed the last phrase implying that they had left the episode behind them, but a number wanted to clarify where they stood by saying that although they had got over it, they had not forgotten, or add a comment such as, '*I don't think about it now, but I'll never forget the worry*'. In spite of the clumsy construction, the question nonetheless added to the picture of women's experiences.

Finally, women in the study were asked whether having the abnormal smear had made them 'think differently about things in any way'. This deliberately general question invited the interviewee to answer in whatever terms she chose. Of those who replied that it had changed the way they thought about things, the most common theme was an awareness of vulnerability and mortality resulting in a re-evaluation of life and a concern not to take one's health for granted. Another common theme was an endorsement of medical developments and screening in particular. The following quotes give a sense of some of the feelings which women expressed at this point (Posner and Vessey, 1988: 73):

> *It's nice to remember what's important and what isn't. I look at life in a slightly different way. In a way, (I) was very lucky — it could have been worse — though at the time it was awful.*

> *They know it's common; they know it's only a small thing. To you — it's the end of the world.*

Allowing the articulation of the lay experience of this medical intervention process revealed important differences between the lay and medical views which needed to be understood in any attempt to minimise the unintended negative consequences of this preventive activity. The report of the study was submitted to the funding body where there was both interest and concern. The concern from one quarter was that possible individual characteristics which supposedly predisposed women to be distressed by the episode should be identified, and that such reactions as described should not be publicised in case other women were alarmed by them[12]. However, the evidence was that women were generally alarmed by an abnormal smear finding in the absence of sufficient information to assess its implications, and reassured by finding that other women had similar reactions to their own at various stages of the subsequent process. A strong motivation for taking part in the study was the idea, often voiced by an interviewee, that by doing so, she could in some way help other women going through the same process, subsequently. Clearly this could only be the case if the study participants' experiences were presented in a form accessible to a wider and relevant audience. It was suggested to the researcher that the King's Fund could be interested in a publication based on the report and indeed this proved to be the case[13]. The report was edited and recommendations for improved practice added. Through this publication and accompanying press attention, as well as presentations to professional audiences, the findings of the study were disseminated and contributed to a growing awareness and understanding of the problem of the 'costs' of cervical screening in terms of the unwanted, unintended effects of the medical intervention process upon women involved.

If women were to experience the abnormality of CIN with less anxiety and conceptualise it with less morbid implications, there was an information gap which needed to be filled. To do so could empower women to go through the process as 'well women', rather than passive patients, taking their full part in the preservation of their own health. There appeared to be, in particular, a need to make available the idea of CIN as a stage between normality and

---

12   *The psychological evidence is that people going through stressful medical procedures are helped by being told details of the procedures and possible pain involved, beforehand. See Johnson J (1983) Preparing patients to cope with stress while hospitalised. In: Wilson-Barnett J (ed) Patient Teaching. Churchill-Livingstone, Edinburgh: pp19–33.*

13   *Posner T and Vessey M (1988) Prevention of Cervical Cancer: The Patient's View. King's Fund, London.*

disease, and the acknowledgement that abnormal cells may not necessarily progress to become a carcinoma, but constitute a risk factor for which intervention is possible, and may be desired. One of the end results of the research process was for the researcher to write an information leaflet for the Women's Health Information Centre (WHIC as it was then, now 'Women's Health')[14], an attempt to bridge the gap between biomedical and ordinary language by supplying accurate information and appropriate words for discussing the condition, and making concepts of risk and prevention processes more accessible, and thus available for the lay person to use in constructing and negotiating her own experience. Other informative leaflets and a helpline followed[15], in recognition of the need for information and support to women in this position.

This chapter has described how survey findings about women's beliefs in relation to cervical screening and cervical cancer were affected by the form of the questions posed, their own experiences and age group, and it has indicated their part in the process of feed-back to health promotion intervention. The subsequent study described was focused on women's experiences of the medical intervention process after an abnormal cervical smear finding, and demonstrated the importance of seeking, understanding and presenting the views of recipients of health care. The study's findings became part of a process encouraging dialogue across the divide between medical views and lay experience in this area of preventive health care.

---

14 *An Abnormal Smear — What Does That Mean? A woman's guide to the medical investigation and treatment of abnormal cervical cells' was produced and distributed by the Women's Health Information Centre, (52 Featherstone Street, London EC1) as Fact Sheet No 2 in 1987.*

15 *The Women's National Cancer Control Campaign produced a leaflet on the cervical smear test and launched their helpline in 1989 to provide breast and cervical screening counselling.*

References

Posner T, Vessey M (1988) *Prevention of Cervical Cancer: The Patient's View*. King's Fund, London

Richard TM *et al* (1980) An analysis of 'long-term' follow-up results in patients with cervical intraepithelial neoplasia treated by cryotherapy. *Am J Obstet Gyn* **137**: 823–6

Richardson AC, Lyon JB (1981) The effect of condom use on squamous cell cervical intraepithelial neoplasia. *Am J Obstet Gyn* **140**(8): 909–13

CHAPTER 10
REFLECTING on the PROCESS and METHODS of RESEARCHING WOMEN'S HEALTH

Linda McKie and Susan Gregory

Introduction

The issues covered in the research projects reported in earlier chapters appear diverse, ranging from infertility, to antenatal services, to services for the adult survivors of sexual abuse (see Table 1, overleaf). The contributors have sought to make visible and audible the views of women and men relevant to the provision of health and health-related services for women. In addition, the reporting of the process and conduct of research in this text has sought to provide realistic portrayals of the difficult choices, resource constraints and power differentials that researchers and respondents must work through. These portrayals stand in opposition to the often idealised presentations of research in many text books.

In this concluding chapter, we draw upon the contributions to the text to consider:

- why start research
- the spectrum of research methods
- approaches to research
- an ethic of practice
- the benefits of health research

- writing up
- feedback and dissemination

Table 10:1 Researching women's health: issues, methods and authors

Health issue	Method(s)	Authors
Antenatal care:	questionnaire	Cochrane
Asian women experiences, responses and views of health services	semi-structured interviews	Bowes and Domokos
Cervical screening services:	discussion groups followed by questionnaire	Gregory and McKie
	population survey in-depth interviews	Posner
Consequences of child sex abuse	questionnaires to adult survivors and statutory bodies delivering services	Gray, Higgs and Pringle
Infertility	un-structured interviews	Wills
Men and pregnancy	semi-structured interviews	Taylor

Why start research?

Research into any topic is undertaken for a number of reasons. If you are a health practitioner, issues regularly arise as a consequence of problems or changes that are part of every day practice. A specific problem may need solving, or background information may offer improvement to diagnosis or care. Frequently, a general interest arising out of personal involvement in an area may drive the enquiry, or it might be an idea for a new direction which has emerged out of past or current work. In addition, many nurses and health care practitioners are undertaking research work as a component of an academic course (see Chapter 1).

For the contributors to this text personal interest or involvement were the main triggers to the development of research Authors have also noted further triggers, including ascertaining and promoting lay views on health needs and services, consideration of service changes, and the development and review of health education material. Commencing research is often a combination of the relevance of the topic to paid employment, participation in an academic course and a review of a service.

The spectrum of methods

In Table 1, the range of methods employed in the research projects were identified. As noted, the projects provide examples of a range of methods and these methods reflect the array available on the spectrum from deductive (quantitative) to inductive (qualitative) approaches. These are outlined in diagrammatic form in Table 2 (ovrleaf).

Quantitative research incorporates standard questions taken to relatively large numbers of people who are selected randomly from the population in question. This may take the form of an interview schedule or questionnaire and may be completed by the respondent or an interviewer. Qualitative research involves in-depth detail which is specific to each case, in the form of semi or unstructured interviews or field observations. The former offers specific answers to specific questions which can be analysed in bulk, usually using a computer programme and this allows claims of

Table 10:2 Some points on the spectrum of methods

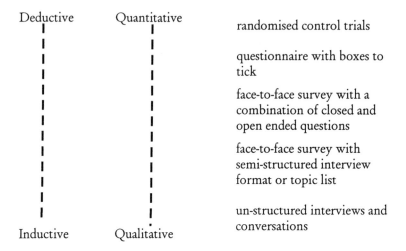

Deductive	Quantitative	
		randomised control trials
		questionnaire with boxes to tick
		face-to-face survey with a combination of closed and open ended questions
		face-to-face survey with semi-structured interview format or topic list
		un-structured interviews and conversations
Inductive	Qualitative	

statistical significance to be made. Important characteristics of this approach are that the study can be replicated and generalised to the population from which the sample has been drawn. Each time the rules governing this approach are broken, or modified, any claims of the results are weakened. The limitations to this approach are that the questions must be the same for all participants. This places limitations on the potential for the respondents to include specific details or definitions of their own that may be important to the understanding of the issue. It also means that sensitive or embarrassing issues may be difficult to enquire into, because this kind of information is often more likely to emerge when respondents use their own ways of expressing themselves. The qualitative approach, conversely, offers the opportunity for respondents to take the time to explore issues in a way they may not have had the chance to previously. This allows complex, sensitive or embarrassing information to emerge which, frequently, not only provides factual information, but also explanations about how that came about. The limitations to this approach are that this kind of data collection is very time consuming and, consequently, it is rare for a study to be able to use other than a small sample. Any claims made about the responses can only be made about the specific respondents, and cannot be generalised to a wider population. Because the enquiry is not a set of standard questions, the comparisons between what is said in terms of similarities and differences can only be the interpretation of the researcher, and cannot be tested statistically.

The notion of a spectrum, from the deductive to the inductive, avoids the binary and often arbitrary distinction between quantitative and qualitative research and the projects reported in this text demonstrate a range of points on such a spectrum. Cochrane (Chapter 6) employed a questionnaire format in her study of ante-natal care with a questionnaire administered on expectations of care and subsequently actual experiences. This method was employed to ensure as wide a coverage of service users as possible in a manner which reflected the limited resources of the project. Gray, Higgs and Pringle (Chapter 7) used two types of questionnaires; one, for the providers of statutory services, employed closed questions for ease of uniformity and comparison between services while a second, for adult survivors of sexual abuse, which made more use of open questions to elicit feelings and views. These choices demonstrate how the questionnaire can be both a deductive and inductive method of collecting data. Grey, Higgs and Pringle also note that their choice of method was, in part, linked to what might be considered as a more appropriate component of a lobbying process with large agencies. Gregory and McKie (Chapter 8), in researching women's views of cervical screening services, employed a questionnaire with many open-ended questions designed as a result of conducting a series of discussion groups and analysing that data. Posner (Chapter 9) contrasts two studies; one a population-based quantitative survey and the other, an in-depth study of the experiences of a series of women experiencing a medical process for the treatment of cervical cell abnormalities. Moving along the spectrum towards the inductive end are a number of studies. Bowes and Domokos (Chapter 4) employed an interview/topic list in interviews with South Asian women. Both Taylor (Chapter 5), men's views on pregnancy, and Wills (Chapter 3), women's views and experiences of infertility, argued that it was important to let respondents speak for themselves and thus they did not develop an interview schedule or topic list. Interviews were unfocused and themes were chosen by the subjects with no assumptions made by the researchers.

Approaches to research

The use of large scale and numerically measurable forms of data collection provide evidence both acceptable and recognisable by the mainstream of both the medical and the academic worlds. However, issues concerned with women's health or women's health responsibilities are frequently best addressed by the use of a qualitative approach, and the majority of our studies follow that path. Qualitative methods tend to be in-depth, one-to-one, small-scale, and in a form that allows the respondent to use her/his own words to describe feelings and experiences. The nature of the enquiry and the feelings of the respondent are often of a sensitive kind, requiring a relaxed and familiar atmosphere, with conditions designed to encourage free and unambiguous disclosure.

On many levels, research in this form cannot fulfil the kind of criteria often demanded of social research. Random sampling would allow the results to claim the representativeness of a wider population. A standard questionnaire, especially one made up of multiple choice answers, would allow direct comparisons between specific and identifiable groups. It would allow tests of statistical significance to be used, to determine whether the results were the consequence of chance, or to chart a pattern of associations and correlations. Nevertheless, small-scale non-numerical data can reveal factors related to women's health issues which may not be predictable early enough to be included in a survey format; factors which may, on the face of it, not have a direct connection with the main health topic under enquiry. A qualitative approach can, within reason, provide the flexibility to allow the researcher to follow a line of investigation not anticipated, and to incorporate new or different languages and communication systems.

A qualitative approach cannot include the range and number of respondents needed for an analysis which produces statistical significance, or allow the opportunity for random sampling. It does, however, provide the chance to identify respondents who demonstrate accurately the characteristics that the research topic requires, allowing all those who do not fulfil that criteria required to be excluded from the study. This accurate identification of information sources ensures that no extraneous factors become drawn into the data set. It is not always easy to identify the people needed for research, who will not necessarily form easily recognisable or identifiable groups. Although a medical issue, whether in terms of services, symptoms or treatments, may be easily identified, the users, or the lifestyles of those users, may not be as clearly or as discretely defined. Even the clarity of symptom definition has been shown to be questionable by, respectively, the infertility and the various cervical screening service studies reported in this text.

An ethic of practice

An important issue implied by all of the studies, and addressed by many feminist researchers (Duelli Klein 1983; Mies 1983; Reinharz 1983), is more ethical than practical or methodological. That is, the level to which the research is 'for' the participants rather than 'about' or 'on' them. This can be reflected in the way in which data are collected — how much is explained about the study to the participants; the opportunities they are offered to use their own language and determine the direction of the enquiry. It may also determine whether participants are offered information about the results, or even invited to take part in the analysis and the writing up. Many of these are not possible, because of the time available for the study, or the requirements of the funding body; because the participants do not wish to take up the offer, or are anonymous and so not connectable. However, if any or all are possible, they provide means by which the place and existence of the participants can be acknowledged, and so contribute to the visibility of women. Research can be designed, as questions can be asked, which either highlight the position of women, or deny it. Thus, the form of the research design is often less important than what is taken for granted within the process of design. For example, Grey, Higgs and Pringle (Chapter 7, p176) in their study of services for people who have been sexually abused, note that the:

> *'personalities, philosophies and backgrounds of researchers can have a major bearing on the way research is shaped and executed.'*

Bowes and Domokos (Chapter 4, p95) further note that the research process may reflect the power differentials between black and white, men and women, researcher and the researched:

> *'...[the researcher] must be alert to the ways in which the interviewing process may reflect this power structure, and what the consequences of this may be.'*

Considering parallels between the worlds of health service and academic research illustrates the unspoken but taken-for-granted understandings that form the structure of these institutions. A fundamental assumption that the power relation between practitioner and patient, between researcher and researched is legitimate and acceptable is rarely challenged. Nevertheless, our studies recommend a more active acknowledgement of the contribution of the patient to the diagnosis of her/his health status through consultation on the views and preferences of the patient. Equally, feminists have drawn attention to the need to ensure the recognition of the contribution of the respondents to the reality of the research results. It is important to identify the values —

invariably patriarchal — which underlie the culture of institutions such as the medical or the academic, as it is to show how women, and female values, are ignored or stereotyped. Taylor (Chapter 5) also identified the exclusion of the male experience of becoming a father from health education materials applicable to pregnancy and childbirth. This further illustrated the cultural stereotyping of roles and experiences, and notions of health needs.

In recognising the power dynamic that exists in most human interactions, medical practitioners and academic researchers must also acknowledge that these relationships are not simple and straight forward. Frequently, the patient will bring with her/him expectations very different from those of the practitioner, just as the respondent constructs her/his own understanding of the research setting. These differing agendas may never be known, and are likely to remain unverbalised. For example, Gregory and McKie (Chapter 8) concluded that women ceased using the cervical smear test service not just when they understood they no longer needed to, but also because they rejected the treatment they had previously received or had heard of from friends and relatives. Most of the studies in the series draw attention to the need for practitioners to look at their own place and role within the health service process (Robert 1985; Roberts 1990).

The benefits of health research

Health and health care services are areas rich with potential for research. The broad range of services offered within the field of health, whether existing or planned, will always require monitoring and evaluation to ensure that their form and focus are, and remain, appropriate and effective. This examination process is important not just for the service itself, but is needed to monitor the conditions within which the service takes place, the attitudes and beliefs of those operating the service, as well as the feelings and experiences of those receiving them.

The beneficiaries of this kind of research should always be the users, whether directly or indirectly. Directly, the results may feed back to them in the form of information and advice offered by the practitioner within the consultation or care process, or in the form of health education and promotion. Indirectly, benefit may be obtained through the improved and extended knowledge gained by the practitioners and the policy makers responsible for the design, construction and process of a specific service. Research results must feed back into the health service process to ensure that each service is efficient and appropriate and offers users the confidence and support needed to encourage it's use.

Women have a special interest in knowing that health services are being monitored and evaluated as a matter of routine. Women are more likely to be involved routinely with health issues in relation to their own reproductive cycles, and they are most likely to act on behalf of children over health matters.

The studies that have formed this text have achieved two aims over and above that of reporting on different aspects of women's health. They have demonstrated the value of focusing specifically on issues that affect women's health and stereotyped perceptions of health and health status, so that attention is drawn to those issues. They have also contributed to a body of knowledge that represents and highlights the experiences of women and men becoming fathers. Even those who do not yet believe that there can be an approach to research which can be justifiably called a feminist methodology have recognised the absence of a gender perspective in much of social research until recent years (Hammersley, 1992). Many feminist researchers have emphasised the necessity for a gender perspective in research in order to raise the visibility of women's experience (Ramazanoglu, 1992; Gelsthorpe, 1992). Bowes and Domokos (p70) further contend that feminist research is about the presentation of differing and potentially competing voices which are rarely heard or recognised; it is the presentation of 'fissured' accounts (Opie, 1992: 58). Despite this aim, they further note that feminist research has paid little attention to issues of 'race' in the research process, and to the relationship between gender issues 'race' issues (Bowes and Domokos, ibid). Wills, in her chapter on women's views and experiences of infertility (Chapter 3), notes that it is important that those participating in research should speak for themselves and meanings should emerge. For Bowes and Domokos (Chapter 4) and Taylor (Chapter 5) this process is not an easy one. Taylor discusses her role and the inherent power differential in being a female researcher working with male respondents on a sensitive topic, men's views of pregnancy. Bowes and Domokos note the differences in experience between the researcher and researched, as one of them, a white researcher, interviewed South Asian women. The authors of these chapters discuss these issues in a frank manner. They present their own 'fissured' accounts of developing and conducting research and thus, they challenge the perceived wisdom in many reports of research which purport an ease and clarity of enquiry which, all too often, is a sanitised version of events.

Writing up

Health research has both process and product elements and the first product of most research is the written account. You cannot begin writing up early enough; field notes, descriptions of project localities, or the services examined can be written up without recourse to the data collection timetable. In fact, the writing begins when you draft the original proposal and should, ideally, continue as you gather material and data. Writing should become joined to the research and one means of securing this is to write up the methods and methodological process at an early stage. This can act as a reflective process ensuring that the realities of the methodological process are considered and represented in the final account. It also provides a draft for a final written account.

Having conducted the research, collected and analysed the relevant materials and data, what next? If you are undertaking research as a component of an academic or post-registration course, there will normally be guidelines on the component sections of any dissertation or thesis. Most sources of funding for research require the production of a report, usually short, concise accounts of the overall results together with a critical account of the methods and methodological approach. If you are starting writing up without guidelines, the following section headings present a possible format (see also Sapsford and Abbott, 1992):

the title; an interesting, explanatory and snappy title is more likely to attract a reader than one which commences 'Further Research On the Views of Women Attending Three Ante-natal Clinics'. Are there key terms/processes in the research? In the case of the example cited, a title might be 'The Views of Women Participating in Ante-natal Care: A Questionnaire Study of Three Clinics'. This title indicates what and who is being researched, and the research method employed;

abstract or summary; an abstract is a short piece of approximately 200 words which outlines the key research questions, the sample, research location(s) and methods, and presents main conclusions. A summary, however, is a more detailed — one to two pages— review of each section of the main report. A short paragraph is normally devoted to outlining the key points of each section;

acknowledgements; it is important to recognise the value of diverse sources of input from amongst people who participated, practitioners and policy makers;

*qualitative research;*sections in the main body of the report might include:

1.   introduction to the research question(s) explaining why these

are relevant or important

2. an explanation about what you did and how

3. data analysis; report the interpretation of data and qualify the reasons for that interpretation

4. report of the results in an easy to follow and read format

5. implications for practice and further research; draw out any implications linking these to evidence presented in previous sections of the report

6. conclusions; review the methods, conduct and major findings

7. appendices; interview schedules, consent forms, practice guidelines etc, might be presented in appendices.

quantitative research; reports of quantitative research only differ from the above as it is necessary to present any statistical analysis of data in an accessible format with an explanation of the actual statistics and the reasons for choosing these.

Central to compiling any written account are the materials and data gathered; it is important to remain in touch with these and review these throughout the writing up process. Writing for journals is a different process and if you are writing for the first time, it is important to seek advice from journal editors and those who have had material published. Some journals are more likely to be read by practitioners in a specific field, e.g. The Nursing Times and Health Education Journal, and will be prepared to consider articles of around 1500 to 3000 words. Other journals, such as the Journal of Advanced Nursing and Health Education Research, Theory and Practice require the study to be located within a consideration of other relevant studies and literature. Articles submitted to these journals should normally demonstrate a consideration of theoretical as well as practice issues. In addition, we would refer readers to a text by Howard Becker (1986) `Writing for Social

Scientists: How to Start and Finish Your Thesis, Book or Article' for a comprehensive guide to writing for a range of audiences.

Feedback and dissemination

Research on women's health cannot be carried out without the respondents actually participating in the process (Roberts, 1992). As Taylor (Chapter 5) demonstrates, researching what are culturally constructed as women's health issues, may also need to take into account the views of men (Roberts, 1981). This presents an interesting dilemma. Oakley (1981) maintains that women are able to appeal to that which they have in common and thus overcome the inequalities between the researcher and researched. Wills (Chapter 3, pp45-6) commented that she employed an approach of conscious partiality, that is the identification with the participants in the study to:

> *'share her experiences as a woman and as a researcher with the participant'.*

Clearly, this may not follow when researching male views and experiences nor the experiences of those who have survived sexual abuse. However, for all of us the research process is a circular one; it starts and finishes with those who give of their time to participate. Contributors to the series were keen to feedback findings to participants and to disseminate project outcomes to respondents, service organisers and providers. Bowes and Domokos (Chapter 4), Cochrane (Chapter 6), Gregory and McKie (Chapter 8), Grey, Higgs and Pringle (Chapter 7) and Posner (Chapter 9) made recommendations to policy makers and service providers, and undertook to bring the data back to the people involved. Taylor (Chapter 5) and Wills (Chapter 3) also made recommendations concerning the design and delivery of health education.

It is pleasing to note that results from a number of the projects are currently being debated by policy makers and service users. The conclusions of the work of Bowes and Domokos (Chapter 4), Cochrane (Chapter 6) and Posner (Chapter 9) add interesting and new insights to their respective areas of study. The chapter by Gray, Higgs and Pringle (Chapter 7) presents material new to many health and social workers.

Conclusions

In this final chapter, we have sought to draw out the many dimensions to the research process as evidenced by contributions to the text. We hope that the series has also demonstrated the value of the research process for those who participated in the projects.

One of our original hopes was that the health care student and professional, busy as they are, might find the contributions to this series accessible and relevant to their work. In addition, we hope that the contributions encourage both students and practitioners to consider the perspective of the people who experience services, directly or indirectly, when designing and conducting research.

References

Becker H (1986) *Writing for Social Scientists: How to Start and Finish Your Thesis, Book or Article*. University of Chicago Press, Chicago

Gelsthorpe L (1992) Response to Martyn Hammersley's paper on feminist methodology. *Sociology* 26(2): 213–8

Hammersley M (1992) On Feminist Methodology. *Sociology* 26(2): 187–206

Duelli Klein R (1983) How to Do What We Want to Do: Thoughts about Feminist Methodology. In: Bowles G, Duelli Klein R eds. *Theories of Women's Studies*. Routledge & Kegan Paul, London

Mies M (1983) Towards a Methodology for Feminist Research. In: Bowles G, Duelli Klein R eds. *Theories of Women's Studies*. Routledge &

Kegan Paul, London

Opie A (1992) Qualitative research; appropriation of the 'other' and empowerment. *Feminist Rev* **40**: 52–69

Ramazanoglu C (1992) On feminist methodology: male reason versus female empowerment. *Sociology* **26**(2): 207–12

Reinharz S (1983) Experiential Analysis: a Contribution to Feminist Research. In: Bowles G, Duelli Klein R eds. *Theories of Women's Studies*. Routledge & Kegan Paul, London

Roberts H (1981) Women and Their Doctors: Power and Powerlessness in the Research Process. In: Roberts H ed., *Doing Feminist Research*. Routledge, London

Roberts H (1985) *The Patient Patients: Women and Their Doctors*. Pandora Press, London

Roberts H ed (1992) *Women's Health Matters*. Routledge, London

Sapsford R, Abbott P (1992) *Research Methods for Nurses and the Caring Professions*. Open University Press, Buckingham

Wolcott H (1990) *Writing Up Qualitative Research*. Sage University Press, London

APPENDIX 1
QUESTIONNAIRE — Adults abused in childhood

Please answer as many questions as you feel able to. It would be helpful if the form was completely filled in, but do not worry if you wish to leave some answers blank.

If the spaces provided are not sufficient to answer questions as you would like, please attach further information.

1   Gender: Male   [ ]   Female   [ ]

2   Age:......................

3   What is your ethnic origin...

4   Are you: Single [ ]   Married [ ]   In a stable
                                                relationship [ ]

5   Do you have an children? Yes [ ]   No [ ]

    If yes, how many ....

    Ages...

    Are they living   at home? [ ]

                          Away [ ]   If away, do   you have access [ ]

6   Are you: Employed   [ ] Nature of Occupation:....................

                    Unemployed [ ] How long? ....

7   Are you in full-time education [ ]   Or part-time education [ ]

8. Who or which of the following would you turn to for emotional help?

    Family   [ ]

    Friends   [ ]

    GP   [ ]

    Other doctor   [ ]

    Social worker   [ ]

    Church   [ ]

    Voluntary agency   [ ]

    Self-help group   [ ]

    Other/please specify...
    ....

9. Were you abused by one person [ ]   More than one [ ]

    Was the abuser a family member [ ]   Outside the family [ ]

    Was the abuser male [ ]   female [ ]   both [ ]

10. Has the abuse stopped Yes [ ]   No [ ]

    If yes, when did it stop?...
    ....
    ....

11. Have you received information about help that is available for people who have been sexually abused?   Yes [ ]   No [ ]

    Where/who did you get it from?....................................

    If you did not take up the help, what prevented you from doing so?...
    ....
    ....
    ....
    ....
    ....

12. a) Did you have help as a child?   [ ]

    b) Did you have help as an adult?   [ ]

    c) Are you having help now?   [ ]

If yes to above from whom did you receive the help as?

a)...

b)...

c)...

		Most	**Least**
Which was the most or least helpful	a)	[ ]	[ ]
	b)	[ ]	[ ]
	c)	[ ]	[ ]

13. Who knew about the abuse?

No one   [ ]

Family member   [ ] Who......................

Friend   [ ]

NSPCC   [ ]

Police   [ ]

Health visitor   [ ]

G P   [ ]

Social services   [ ]

Church   [ ]

Voluntary agency   [ ] Which........................

Teacher/Tutor   [ ]

Other...

14. How did they find out?...
....
....

15. Were legal proceedings started? Yes/No a) to protect you

                                                                    b) prosecute the abuser

    If yes to above what was the outcome?.....................................
    ....
    ....

    If no to above — if you know why please describe:...................
    ....
    ....

Thinking back on your own experience, the answers and comments on the following questions would be of help in planning and lobbying for future services.

Would you prefer to receive help from:

1) A professional agency [ ]   A voluntary/self-help organisation [ ]

2) A male   [ ]   A female [ ]

3) Someone within your   outside your
   community   [ ]   community   [ ]

4) Someone who had been abused themselves [ ]   or not [ ]

5) Similar age [ ]   Older [ ]   Younger [ ]

Which of the following would be helpful to you:

i)   Open acess   [ ]

ii)   Regular appointment times   [ ]

iii) You receive help for as long as **you** think you need it   [ ]

iv)   Group work   [ ]

v)   Individual   [ ]

vi)   Family work   [ ]

vii) 24-Hour phone line   [ ]

viii)   Total confidentiality   [ ]

ix)   Support outside the therapy   [ ]

x)   Setting —   own home   [ ]   away from home [ ]

xi)   Having a support person with you during your
therapy/counselling sessions   [ ]

xii)   Help available for family   [ ]   partners   [ ]   friends [ ]

**We would appreciate any further comments or suggestions that
you would like to make:**

....
....
....
....
....
....
....
....
....
....
....
....
....
....
....
....
....
....

APPENDIX II
C.A.L.L. QUESTIONNAIRE

Dear colleague

C.A.L.L is a voluntary organisation in the north of England with professional supports which seek to fill gaps in provision for those affected by sexual abuse. In conjunction with myself and several other professional consultants, C.A.L.L. is also seeking to develop a research function. Therapeutic services provided by professional and voluntary organisations in the field of sexual bause in this region to an extent seem scattered. To enhance the service to users, we are seeking to carry out an audit of facilities within the northern region in the hope of:

a) developing a wider network of resources

b) targeting for development services which have not yet been provided

c) highlighting training which you feel would benefit service providers, both voluntary and professional.

As a result of that objective we are sending this questionnaire to as many service co-ordinators/managers as possible in the north east region, covering provision, such as health, education, social work, probation and the voluntary/independent sectors.

The questionnaire is divided into three sections: one relating to services in the area of children who have been sexually abused; the second to services relating to adults who have been abused in childhood; the third to adults abused within adulthood.

Lists of potential service users are provided. We are asking you to note:

a) the users to whom you offer resources/services (a simple tick in the appropriate section will usually suffice)

b) what precise age groups are catered for in that user class (for instance, if you have services for male children who have been abused, are there age limits on that provision?)

c) which professional or non-professional personnel provide those services (e.g. social workers or clinical psychologists etc)

d) what form that provision takes, i.e. is it Individual counselling and/or Groupwork provision and/or Family-centred provision (you should enter I and/or G and/or F as appropriate in the space provided).

We recognise that you are extremely busy but we hope you will find time for the questionnaire in the interests of the users whom we all service.

Thank you very much for your assistance.

On completion, please return the questionnaire to myself at the address on the letterhead. However, I would be grateful if you could direct any queries to SHARON GRAY on the following telephone number:

Yours sincerely

KEITH PRINGLE

SENIOR LECTURER IN SOCIAL WORK

SCHOOL OF SOCIAL AND INTERNATIONAL STUDIES

UNIVERSITY OF SUNDERLAND

C.A.L.L. QUESTIONNAIRE

Circulation to as many service provision managers/co-ordinators as possible in the north east region including: **voluntary/self-help services; health service managers** (e.g. unit managers, heads of clin. psych., cons. psychiatrists, cons. paediatricians, heads of community services), GPs; **education service managers** (e.g. heads of schools, of ed. psych. services, of 'special units', ed. welfare services, ch. guidance units); **heads of social work services** (e.g. field services. res. services, hospital S.W services, vol/independent S.W. services); **probation services.**

Voluntary Groups:

Health Service:

Education Service:

Social Service

Probation Service:

If you are aware of any other agencies/ organisations in the region working with the issue of sexual abuse, we would be most grateful if you would let us have details
here...
....
....
....

NAME.......................... ORGANISATION....................................

POST..

SERVICES IN RELATION TO CHILDREN WHO HAVE BEEN ABUSED

	Ages	Who provides	Type of provision I and/or G and/or F
Male abused			
Female abused			
Male abuser			
Female abuser			
Non-abusing parent			
Siblings of abused			
Extended family			
Close friends of abused			
Family of abuser			

Could you please also give here details of any preventative work done in your area of provision — could you please say whether it is aimed at those who may be abused or at those who are at risk of abusing..

....

....

Do you make particular provision of services for people who are black or from an ethnic minority group in any of the categories in the grid on the previous page? If so, please specify.......................................

....

....

....

Any other comments or details which you wish to mention...............

....

....

....

SERVICES IN RELATION TO ADULTS WHO HAVE BEEN SEXUALLY ABUSED IN CHILDHOOD

	Ages	Who provides	Type of provision I and/or G and/or F
Male abused			
Female abused			
Male abuser			
Female abuser			
Non-abusing parent			
Siblings of abused			
Extended family			
Close friends of abused			
Family of abuser			

Please give details of any preventative work carried out in your area of provision and at whom it is targeted..
....
....

Do you make particular provision of services for people who are black or from an ethnic minority group in any of the categories in the grid on the previous page? If so, please specify....................................
....
....
....

Any other comments or details you wish to give...................................
....
....
....

SERVICES IN RELATION TO ADULTS WHO HAVE BEEN SEXUALLY ABUSED IN ADULTHOOD

	Ages	Who provides	Type of provision I and/or G and/or F
Male abused			
Female abused			
Male abuser			
Female abuser			
Non-abusing parent			
Siblings of abused			
Extended family			
Close friends of abused			
Family of abuser			

Please give details of any preventative work carried out in your area of provision and at whom it is targeted...
....
....

Do you make particular provision of services for people who are black or from an ethnic minority group in any of the categories in the grid on the previous page? If so, please specify..................................
....
....
....

Any other comments or details you wish to give................................
....
....
....

GENERAL QUESTIONS

1   Does your service base its work on any particular theoretical framework or philosophy — if so, which?

2.   Finally, if you wish to do so, please state here any number and relevant training needs which would benefit you or your staff in providing a service to users

THANK YOU VERY MUCH INDEED

Index